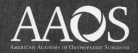

M000159644

Bloodborne and Airborne Pathogens

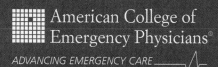
American College of
Emergency Physicians®
ADVANCING EMERGENCY CARE

EIGHTH EDITION

Medical Writers

Robin E. Bishop, MS, MICP, CHS III, EMP, MEP, DOIC

Andrew Bartkus, MSN, JD, RN, CEN, CCRN, CFRN, NRP, Esq.

Medical Editors

Alfonso Mejia, MD, MPH, FAAOS

Jacqueline A. Nemer, MD, FACEP

Bob Elling, MPA, EMT-P

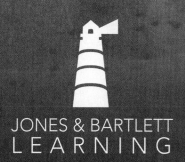

JONES & BARTLETT
LEARNING

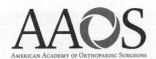
AMERICAN ACADEMY OF ORTHOPAEDIC SURGEONS

Substantial discounts on bulk quantities of Jones & Bartlett Learning publications are available to corporations, professional associations, and other qualified organizations. For details and specific discount information, contact the special sales department at Jones & Bartlett Learning via the above contact information or send an email to specialsales@jblearning.com.

Jones & Bartlett Learning books and products are available through most bookstores and online booksellers. To contact the Jones & Bartlett Learning Public Safety Group directly, call 800-832-0034, fax 978-443-8000, or visit our website, www.psglearning.com.

Production Credits
VP, Product Development: Christine Emerton
Director of Product Management: Jonathan Epstein
Product Manager: Carly Mahoney
Content Strategist: Ashley Procum
Project Manager: Jessica DeMartin
Project Specialist: John Coakley
Digital Project Specialist: Angela Dooley
Director of Marketing Operations: Brian Rooney
VP, Sales, Public Safety Group: Matthew Maniscalco
Content Services Manager: Colleen Lamy

VP, Manufacturing and Inventory Control: Therese Connell
Composition: S4Carlisle Publishing Services
Project Management: S4Carlisle Publishing Services
Cover and Text Design: Scott Moden
Senior Media Development Editor: Troy Liston
Rights & Permissions Manager: John Rusk
Rights Specialist: Liz Kincaid
Cover Image: © Dr. P. Marazzi/Science Source
Printing and Binding: LSC Communications

Library of Congress Cataloging-in-Publication Data
Names: Bishop, Robin E., author. | Bartkus, Andrew, author. | American Academy of Orthopaedic Surgeons, author.
Title: Bloodborne and airborne pathogens / Robin Bishop, Drew Bartkus, AAOS.
Description: Eighth edition. | Burlington, Massachusetts : Jones & Bartlett Learning, [2022] | Preceded by Bloodborne and airborne pathogens / [edited by] Benjamin Gulli, Keith Borg, Robin E. Bishop. Seventh edtion. [2018.] | Includes bibliographical references and index.
Identifiers: LCCN 2020058566 | ISBN 9781284232288 (paperback)
Subjects: MESH: Blood-Borne Pathogens | Communicable Disease Control | Occupational Diseases—prevention & control | Health Personnel
Classification: LCC RA642.B56 | NLM WA 790 | DDC 614.4/4—dc23
LC record available at https://lccn.loc.gov/2020058566

6048

Printed in the United States of America
25 24 23   10 9 8 7 6 5 4 3

Contents

Welcome to the Emergency Care & Safety Institute

Welcome to the Emergency Care & Safety Institute (ECSI), brought to you by the American Academy of Orthopaedic Surgeons (AAOS) and the American College of Emergency Physicians (ACEP).

ECSI is an internationally renowned organization that provides training and certifications that meet job-related requirements as defined by regulatory authorities such as the Occupational Safety and Health Administration (OSHA), The Joint Commission, and state offices of EMS, Education, Transportation, and Health. Our courses are delivered throughout a range of industries and markets worldwide, including colleges and universities, business and industry, government, public safety agencies, hospitals, private training companies, and secondary school systems.

ECSI programs are offered in association with the AAOS and ACEP. AAOS, the world's largest medical organization of musculoskeletal specialists, is known as the original name in EMS publishing with the first EMS textbook ever in 1971, and ACEP is widely recognized as the leading name in all of emergency medicine.

ECSI Course Catalog

Individuals seeking training from ECSI can choose from among various traditional classroom-based courses or alternative online courses such as:

- Advanced Cardiac Life Support (ACLS)
- Babysitter Safety
- Basic Life Support (BLS) for Health Care Providers
- CPR and AED
- Bloodborne and Airborne Pathogens
- Driver Safety
- First Aid (standard, advanced, pediatric, wilderness, sports, pet)
- And more!

ECSI offers a wide range of textbooks, instructor and student support materials, and interactive technology, including online courses. ECSI student manuals are the center of an integrated teaching and learning system that offers resources to better support instructors and train students. The instructor supplements provide practical hands-on, time-saving tools like PowerPoint presentations, skills demonstration videos, and web-based distance learning resources. Technology resources provide interactive exercises and simulations to help students become prepared for any emergency.

Documents attesting to ECSI's recognitions of satisfactory course completion will be issued to those who successfully meet the course requirements. Written acknowledgment of a participant's successful course completion is provided in the form of a Course Completion Card, issued by the ECSI.

Visit **www.ECSInstitute.org** today!

Acknowledgments

The medical writers, medical editors, Jones & Bartlett Learning Public Safety Group, American Academy of Orthopaedic Surgeons, and American College of Emergency Physicians would like to thank all of the reviewers who generously offered their time, expertise, and talent to the making of this eighth edition.

Reviewers

Petra M. Bergenthal, BSN, RN, CIC
University of New Mexico
Sandoval Regional Medical Center
Rio Rancho, New Mexico

Erick Arden Bourassa, PhD, MD
Mississippi College
Clinton, Mississippi

Sean J. Britton, MPA, NRP, CPHQ
United Health Services Hospitals
Superior Ambulance Service
Binghamton, New York

Kent Courtney
Paramedic, Fire Fighter, Rescue Technician,
    Educator
Essential Safety Training and Consulting
Lake Montezuma, Arizona

James E. Gretz, BS, NRP, CCP-C
JeffSTAT Education Center
Thomas Jefferson University Hospital
Philadelphia, Pennsylvania

William Paul McKinney, MD, FACP
Professor and Associate Dean for Research
University of Louisville School of Public Health
    and Information Services
Louisville, Kentucky

Jennifer TeWinkel Shea, MBA, AEMT
Regions Hospital
St. Paul, Minnesota

Steve Trala, RN, MPH, MSN, CFRN, NRP
University of Vermont Medical Center
Burlington, Vermont

Christopher C. Williams, PhD, NRP
Guilford County EMS
Greensboro, North Carolina

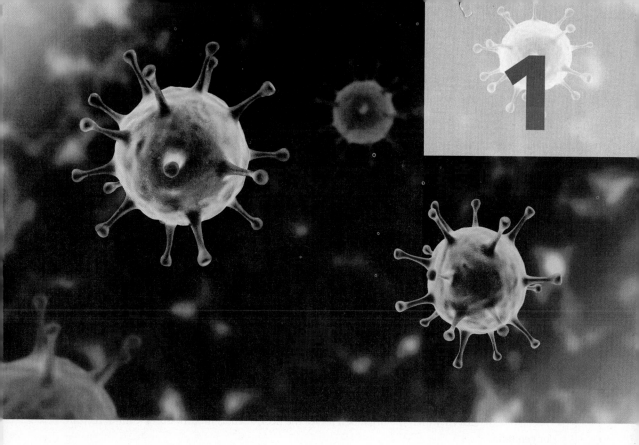

Introduction

What Are Pathogens?

A **pathogen** is any microorganism that produces disease. There are several types of disease-causing pathogens commonly encountered in the occupational setting. These include viruses (eg, measles), bacteria (eg, tuberculosis), fungi (eg, athlete's foot), protozoa (eg, giardiasis), prions (eg, mad cow disease), parasitic worms (eg, tapeworms), and rickettsia (eg, typhus and Rocky Mountain spotted fever).

What Are Bloodborne Pathogens?

Bloodborne pathogens are disease-causing microorganisms (such as viruses, bacteria, or parasites) carried in the **blood**. Common bloodborne pathogens include the **hepatitis B virus**

(HBV), hepatitis C virus (HCV), and human immunodeficiency virus (HIV). These pathogens may be transmitted through contact with contaminated blood or body fluids.

What Are Airborne Pathogens?

Airborne pathogens are disease-causing agents that spread infection through mechanisms such as droplets, dust, and smaller aerosolized particles or drops. These agents travel through the air from person to person or become deposited onto a surface and eventually reach another susceptible person. For example, the common cold travels directly from person to person by coughing and sneezing. As you read this text, it is important not to confuse the term "airborne pathogen," meaning may travel in/through the air, with the concept of "airborne isolation" and the "airborne infection isolation room." The latter two terms have evolved in health care to refer to the measures required to protect health care providers from being exposed to tiny aerosolized particles capable of remaining suspended in the air for long periods of time or traveling great distances while defying gravity.

Chain of Transmission

Several elements must exist for a pathogen to cause illness or disease. These elements are referred to as the chain of transmission. The chain includes:

- Reservoir: An infected human, animal, plant, soil, water, or other substance in which an infectious agent can survive and reproduce.
- Portal of exit: Exit by which the organism leaves the host, such as mouth, nose, wound, rectum, or genitalia.
- Route of transmission: Mechanism by which the disease is spread, such as contact, air or droplet, food, or vector.
- Portal of entry: Opening by which the organism enters the host, such as mouth, nose, wound, rectum, genitalia, or nonintact skin.
- Susceptible host: Anyone, including you.

When referring to occupational disease transmission, the term *exposure* includes all the elements in the chain of transmission except for the susceptible host. Thus, an exposure indicates that blood or other potentially infectious materials (OPIMs) (whether infected or not) entered a host portal of entry. Common portals of entry are mucous membranes and nonintact skin. Mucous membranes are areas of the body, other than the skin, that are exposed to the outside environment. These areas have a lining of specialized epithelial cells that prevent harmful pathogens and other substances from entering the body. Mucous membranes include the eyes, digestive tract, urinary tract, respiratory tract, vagina, and the inside of the ears. An exposure does not necessarily result in infection because of the variation in host immunity and concentration of pathogens in an exposure. More details regarding exposure, routes of transmission, and prevention measures will be discussed in later chapters.

Pathogens and the Law

Because certain occupations may involve contact with blood or OPIMs, the US Department of Labor's Occupational Safety and Health Administration (OSHA) has issued regulations to reduce or eliminate employee exposure to bloodborne and airborne (respiratory) pathogens. These regulations, known as the OSHA Bloodborne Pathogens Standard (29 CFR 1910.1030) **FIGURE 1-1** and Respiratory Protection Standard (29 CFR 1910.134), are designed to promote employee safety through proper training,

OSHA Bloodborne Pathogens Standard

OSHA Bloodborne Pathogens Regulations Section 1910.1030

Part 1910-[Amended]

Subpart Z-[Amended]

1. The general authority citation for subpart Z of 29 CFR part 1910 continues to read as follows and a new citation for 1910.1030 is added:

Authority: Secs. 6 and 8, Occupational Safety and Health Act, 29 U.S.C. 655, 657, Secretary of Labor's Orders Nos. 12-71 (36 CFR 8754), 8-76 (41 CFR 25059), or 9-83 (48 CFR 35736), as applicable; and 29 CFR part 1911.

*   *   *

Section 1910.1030 also issued under 29 U.S.C. 853.

*   *   *

2. Section 1910.1030 is added to read as follows:

1910.1030 Bloodborne Pathogens.

(a) Scope and Application

This section applies to all occupational exposure to blood or other potentially infectious materials as defined by paragraph (b) of this section.

(b) Definitions

For purposes of this section, the following shall apply:

Assistant Secretary means the Assistant Secretary of Labor for Occupational Safety and Health, or designated representative.

Blood means human blood, human blood components, and products made from human blood.

Bloodborne Pathogens means pathogenic microorganisms that are present in human blood and can cause disease in humans. These pathogens include, but are not limited to, Hepatitis B Virus [HBV] and Human Immunodeficiency Virus [HIV].

Clinical Laboratory means a workplace where diagnostic or other screening procedures are performed on blood or other potentially infectious materials.

Contaminated means the presence or the reasonably anticipated presence of blood or other potentially infectious materials on an item or surface.

Contaminated Laundry means laundry which has been soiled with blood or other potentially infectious materials or may contain sharps.

Contaminated Sharps means any contaminated object that can penetrate the skin including, but not limited to, needles, scalpels, broken glass, broken capillary tubes, and exposed ends of dental wires.

Decontamination means the use of physical or chemical means to remove, inactivate, or destroy bloodborne pathogens on a surface or item to the point where they are no longer capable of transmitting infectious particles and the surface or item is rendered safe for handling, use, or disposal.

Director means the Director of the National Institute for Occupational Safety and Health, U.S. Department of Health and Human Services, or designated representative.

Engineering Controls means controls (e.g., sharps disposal containers, self-sheathing needles) that isolate or remove the bloodborne pathogens hazard from the workplace.

Exposure Incident means a specific eye, mouth, other mucous membrane, non-intact skin, or parenteral contact with blood or other potentially infectious materials that results from the performance of an employee's duties.

Handwashing Facilities means a facility providing an adequate supply of running potable water, soap, and single use towels or hot air drying machines.

Licensed Health Care Professional is a person whose legally permitted scope of practice allows him or her to independently perform the activities required by paragraph (f) Hepatitis B vaccination and Post-Exposure Evaluation and Follow-Up.

HBV means Hepatitis B Virus.

HIV means Human Immunodeficiency Virus.

Occupational Exposure means reasonably anticipated skin, eye, mucous membrane, or parenteral contact with blood or other potentially infectious materials that may result from the performance of an employee's duties.

Other Potentially Infectious Materials means

(1) The following human body fluids: semen, vaginal secretions, cerebrospinal fluid, synovial fluid, pleural fluid, pericardial fluid, peritoneal fluid, amniotic fluid, saliva in dental procedures, any body fluid that is visibly contaminated with blood, and all body fluids in situations where it is difficult or impossible to differentiate between body fluids;

(2) Any unfixed tissue or organ (other than intact skin) from a human (living or dead); and

(3) HIV-containing cell or tissue cultures, organ cultures, and HIV- or HBV-containing culture medium or other solutions; and blood, organs, or other tissues from experimental animals infected with HIV or HBV.

Parenteral means piercing mucous membranes or the skin barrier through such events as needlesticks, human bites, cuts, and abrasions.

FIGURE 1-1 Occupational Safety and Health Administration (OSHA) Bloodborne Pathogens Standard.

education, safety, prevention, and exposure control measures. OSHA is often confused with the National Institute for Occupational Safety and Health (NIOSH). NIOSH is a research and educational entity within the United States Centers for Disease Control and Prevention (CDC) focused on reducing worker illnesses and injuries. Even though both OSHA and NIOSH have similar goals, NIOSH does not enforce regulations or laws related to worker safety.

CAL/OSHA

Cal/OSHA is the California Occupational Safety and Health Administration, which is responsible for ensuring the safety and health of California employees. Throughout the text, California participants may wish to refer to the boxes, which indicate Cal/OSHA Standards that differ from federal OSHA requirements. Other states and political jurisdictions may have similar regulations that surpass OSHA. You should become familiar with any additional regulations that might affect your agency or employer.

FYI

The OSHA Respiratory Protection Standard (29 CFR 1910.134) and the Bloodborne Pathogens Standard (29 CFR 1910.1030) can be found in the accompanying online resources.

FYI

California has an additional requirement known as the Aerosol Transmissible Disease Standard (California Code of Regulations, Title 8, Section 5199).

Meeting OSHA Standards

The goal of this training is to educate employees regarding various pathogens and how to minimize or eliminate exposure to pathogens by using standard precautions, transmission-based precautions, personal protective equipment (PPE), administrative controls, work practice controls, and engineering controls. This multilayered combination provides the best approach to maintaining pathogen safety in the workplace.

OSHA

OSHA requires all employers (who are covered in the Bloodborne Pathogens Standard 1910.1030) to offer postexposure evaluation, exposure reporting, confidential medical evaluation, postexposure prophylaxis, counseling, and follow-up treatment to any employee who experiences an exposure incident at work.

Who Needs OSHA Training?

Employees who are required to handle human blood or OPIMs must receive training in various pathogens as well as on-site training to implement the requirements of specific work environments properly. OSHA requires that employees have access to a copy of the OSHA Bloodborne Pathogens and Respiratory Protection Standards. The Standards list several elements of information that must be covered in employees' training.

The scope of the Standards is not limited to employees with job descriptions that include expected, direct occupational exposure to blood and OPIMs. The Standards also address employees with the potential for exposure, not just actual exposure. These employees, such as those trained in first aid and identified by their employers as being responsible for administering medical assistance on the job, do need to receive training in accordance with the OSHA Standards. For example, emergency department intake personnel (eg, registration staff) may not have an actual exposure to a bleeding patient, but the potential for exposure still exists.

> **OSHA**
>
> Records that document employee training assist the employer and OSHA in determining whether the training program adequately addresses the risks involved in each job.

Employees

Any employee who has occupational exposure to blood or OPIMs is included within the scope of the Standards. This includes part-time, temporary health care workers known as "per diem" employees and volunteers.

All employees initially assigned to tasks with potential for occupational exposure to blood or OPIMs must receive training on the hazards associated with blood and OPIMs **FIGURE 1-2**. Protective measures to minimize the risk of occupational exposure must also be reviewed in each training.

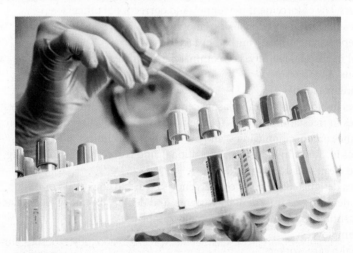

FIGURE 1-2 Any employee who has potential for occupational exposure to blood or OPIMs is required to receive training.
© Romaset/Shutterstock.

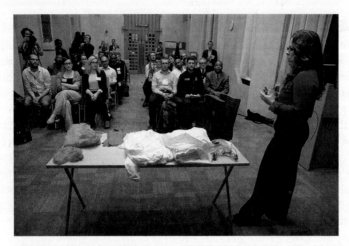

FIGURE 1-3 Annual training is necessary to ensure employee safety.
© WPA Pool/Getty Images News/Getty Images.

Training is offered at least annually and must be provided within 1 year of the original training **FIGURE 1-3**. Whenever a change in responsibilities, procedures, or work situation affects an employee's occupational exposure, additional training, or as stated in the Standard, "retraining," must take place. Retraining is more specific than annual training. For example, retraining must occur when new equipment is brought to the worksite that might affect the employee's potential exposure to pathogens.

The following job classifications may be associated with tasks that have occupational exposure to blood or OPIMs, but the Standard is not limited to employees in these positions:

- Physicians, physicians' assistants, nurses, nurse practitioners, and other health care employees in clinics, hospitals, and physicians' offices
- Emergency medical responders, emergency medical technicians, advanced emergency medical technicians, paramedics, and other emergency medical service providers
- Firefighters, law enforcement personnel, and correctional officers
- Employees of clinical and diagnostic laboratories
- Housekeepers in health care and other facilities
- Personnel in hospital laundries or commercial laundries that service health care or public safety institutions
- Tissue bank personnel
- Employees in blood banks and plasma centers who collect, transport, and test blood
- Employees in freestanding clinics (eg, hemodialysis clinics, urgent care clinics, health maintenance organization clinics, and family planning clinics)
- Employees in clinics in industrial, educational, and correctional facilities (eg, those who collect blood and clean and dress wounds)
- Employees designated to provide emergency first aid to coworkers or others
- Dentists, dental hygienists, dental assistants, and dental laboratory technicians
- Staff of institutions for the developmentally disabled
- Hospice employees
- Home health care workers
- Staff of nursing homes and long-term care facilities

- Employees of funeral homes and mortuaries
- HIV and HBV research laboratory and production facility workers
- Employees handling regulated waste or sharps, such as custodial workers required to clean up contaminated sharps or spills of blood or OPIMs
- Medical equipment service and repair personnel
- Maintenance workers (eg, plumbers) in health care facilities and employees of substance abuse clinics

Why Do I Need This Manual?

This manual will not make you an expert in bloodborne or airborne pathogens or the treatment of diseases caused by these pathogens. The manual does give you important and necessary information as required by the OSHA Bloodborne Pathogens Standard and Respiratory Protection Standard. Your instructor may expand on the information according to worksite-specific practices.

This manual provides OSHA-specific bloodborne and airborne transmissible pathogens guidelines and is used with your worksite-specific training. You are encouraged to gather worksite-specific details on various work pages throughout the manual. Exercises at the end of each chapter help you check what you have learned and understand how it may be applied to your particular worksite requirements.

FYI

The employer must maintain records in a way that segregates sharps injuries from other types of work-related injuries in a sharps injury log.

Site-Specific Work Page
Employee Training

Your name: _____

Date/Time of training: _____

Training location: _____

This bloodborne pathogen training has been conducted by: _____

Attach a few comments about their qualifications.

_____

_____

Name of your supervisor or other responsible person you would contact in the event of an exposure:

_____

Bloodborne pathogen training materials are available at: _____

This is:

     Initial training: ❑ Yes   ❑ No

     Retraining: ❑ Yes   ❑ No

     Annual training: ❑ Yes   ❑ No

This training occurred during my routine work hours: ❑ Yes   ❑ No

This training occurred at no cost to me: ❑ Yes   ❑ No

A copy of the Standards is included in my pathogens manual: ❑ Yes   ❑ No

The training materials are easy for me to understand: ❑ Yes   ❑ No

The training materials are in a language I understand: ❑ Yes   ❑ No

Terms are defined in my pathogens manual: ❑ Yes   ❑ No

My company's exposure control plan is available at: _____

Training records are available for 3 years and are kept by: _____

I may request a copy of my training record from: _____

Request for a copy of my training record is to be provided within 15 days: ❏ Yes   ❏ No

Training records are considered confidential: ❏ Yes   ❏ No

Questions about the Standards were answered by the trainer: ❏ Yes   ❏ No

My questions about the OSHA Standards are:_____

_____

PREP KIT

Vital Vocabulary

administrative controls Standard operating procedures and policies that prevent exposures. These include developing training programs, enforcing exclusion of ill employees, implementing respiratory hygiene/cough etiquette strategies, promoting and providing vaccinations, and developing exposure control plans.

airborne pathogens Disease-causing agents that spread infection through mechanisms such as droplets or dust.

blood The term *blood* refers to human blood, human blood components (which include plasma, platelets, and serosanguinous fluids), and medications derived from blood (such as immunoglobulins, albumin, and clotting factors VIII and IX).

bloodborne pathogens Disease-causing microorganisms that are carried in human blood or other potentially infectious materials. These pathogens include, but are not limited to, hepatitis B virus, hepatitis C virus, and human immunodeficiency virus.

contaminated sharps Any contaminated object that can penetrate the skin including, but not limited to, needles, scalpels, broken capillary tubes, and exposed ends of dental wires.

engineering controls Techniques for removal or isolation of a workplace hazard through technology. An airbone infection isolation room, a protective environment, engineered sharps injury prevention devices, and sharps containers are examples of engineering controls.

exposure incident A specific eye, mouth, mucous membrane, nonintact skin, or parenteral contact with blood or OPIMs that results from the performance of an employee's duties.

hepatitis B virus (HBV) A virus that causes liver infection. It ranges in severity from a mild illness lasting a few weeks (acute) to a serious long-term (chronic) illness that can lead to liver disease or liver cancer.

hepatitis C virus (HCV) A virus that causes liver infection. HCV infection sometimes results in an acute illness but most often becomes a chronic condition that can lead to cirrhosis of the liver and liver cancer.

human immunodeficiency virus (HIV) A virus that infects immune system blood cells in humans and renders them less effective in preventing disease.

mucous membrane An area of the body, other than the skin, that is exposed to the outside environment. These areas have specialized epithelial cells that prevent pathogens and other materials from entering the body. Mucous membranes include the respiratory tract, digestive tract, urinary tract, vagina, eyes, and inside of the ear.

occupational exposure Reasonably anticipated skin, eye, mucous membrane, or parenteral contact with blood or other potentially infectious materials (OPIMs) that may result from the performance of an employee's duties. "Reasonably anticipated contact" includes, among others, contact with blood or OPIMs (including regulated waste) as well as incidents of needlesticks.

other potentially infectious material (OPIM) Fluids such as semen, vaginal secretions, cerebrospinal fluid, synovial fluid, pleural fluid, pericardial fluid, peritoneal fluid, amniotic fluid, saliva in dental procedures, any body fluid that is visibly contaminated with blood, and all body fluids in situations where it is difficult or impossible to differentiate between body fluids; any unfixed tissue or

PREP KIT continued

organ (other than intact skin) from a live or dead human; any cell and tissue cultures, and human immunodeficiency virus (HIV)- or hepatitis B virus (HBV)-containing culture medium or other solutions; and blood, organs, or other tissues from experimental animals (especially those infected with HIV or HBV).

pathogen Any microorganism that causes disease.

personal protective equipment (PPE) A variety of barriers used alone or in combination to protect mucous membranes, skin, and clothing from contact with infectious agents. PPE includes gloves, masks, respirators, goggles, face shields, and gowns.

regulated waste Liquid or semiliquid blood or other potentially infectious materials (OPIMs); contaminated items that would release blood or OPIMs in a liquid or semiliquid state if compressed; items that are caked with dried blood or OPIMs and are capable of releasing these materials during handling; contaminated sharps; and pathological and microbiological wastes containing blood or OPIMs.

sharps Any objects used or encountered in the industries covered by subsection (a) of the Occupational Safety and Health Administration Bloodborne Pathogens Standard that can be reasonably anticipated to penetrate the skin or any other part of the body and to result in an exposure incident. These objects include, but are not limited to, needle devices, scalpels, lancets, broken glass, broken capillary tubes, exposed ends of dental wires and dental knives, drills, and burs.

sharps injury Any injury caused by a sharp, including, but not limited to, cuts, abrasions, or needlesticks.

sharps injury log A written or electronic record satisfying the requirements of subsection (c)(2) of the Occupational Safety and Health Administration Bloodborne Pathogens Standard.

standard precautions A group of infection prevention practices that apply to all patients, regardless of suspected or confirmed diagnosis or presumed infection status.

transmission-based precautions Additional steps instituted when routes of transmission are not interrupted by standard precautions alone; that is, contact precautions, droplet precautions, airborne precautions.

work practice controls Controls that reduce the likelihood of exposure by altering the manner in which a task is performed (eg, prohibiting recapping of needles by a two-handed technique and use of patient handling techniques).

Check Your Knowledge

1. What type of task would require training in bloodborne pathogens and OPIM safety?

2. If there is a change to my work practices that would alter my exposure to bloodborne pathogens, I would receive retraining.

  A. True   **B.** False

3. I must receive training every year.

  A. True

  B. False

4. Employers do not need to maintain records in a way that segregates sharps injuries from other types of work-related injuries.

   A. True

   B. False

5. Part-time employees and volunteers are not covered under the Standards.

   A. True

   B. False

6. All exposures result in infection.

   A. True

   B. False

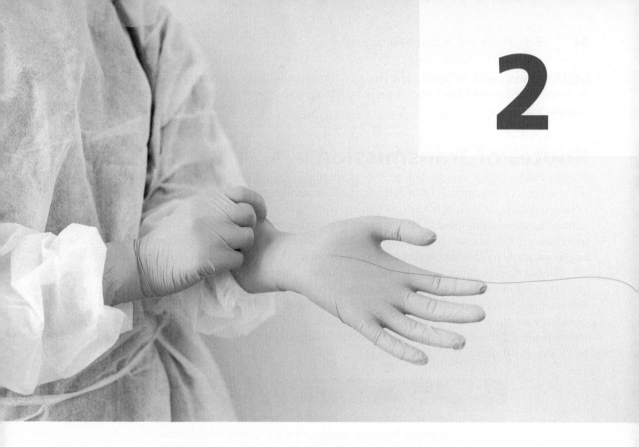

2

Prevention Strategies

Overview

The Occupational Safety and Health Administration (OSHA) and the Centers for Disease Control and Prevention (CDC) have identified several strategies to prevent or reduce exposure to bloodborne pathogens and other potentially infectious materials (OPIMs). The likelihood of becoming infected after a single exposure to a pathogen depends on a variety of factors. The factors most often associated with transmission of disease include the presence of the pathogen in the source blood or OPIM, the type of injury or contact (eg, splash or puncture wound), the pathogen level present in the source individual (patient), the host's current health (eg, immunocompromised), and vaccination status. The point of the strategies is to eliminate or reduce the contribution of these factors to pathogen transmission. Thus,

OSHA mandates seek to "break" the chain of transmission at one or more points along the chain. In order to understand the value of these mandates, one must first understand how pathogens are transmitted.

Routes of Transmission

The five main routes of transmission are contact, droplet, air, food, and vector. Vector (nonhuman) transmission occurs when animals or insects (eg, fleas, mosquitoes, birds, rodents) transmit pathogens, such as rabies, malaria, or West Nile virus, to human hosts. Pathogens primarily transmitted through food are outside the scope of this manual. Vector-transmitted pathogens that may also be transmitted from human to human will be addressed briefly in later sections. The key to infection prevention in the occupational setting primarily revolves around interrupting the contact, droplet, and airborne transmission routes.

Contact transmission is the most common. Contact transmission can be further classified into direct contact or indirect contact. Direct contact occurs when a pathogen is transmitted from person to person. For example, direct contact transmission may occur when a person with nonintact skin on the hands does not wear gloves while rendering care to a patient with an open, bleeding wound. Indirect contact transmission occurs when a person is exposed to pathogens on fomites (contaminated objects), such as bed linens, instruments, and soiled dressings.

CAL/OSHA

Cal/OSHA requires not only the hepatitis B vaccination but also several other vaccinations, including measles, mumps, rubella, and seasonal influenza, listed in the Aerosol Transmissible Disease Standard (California Code of Regulations, Title 8, Section 5199).

Droplet transmission occurs when droplets contaminated with infectious pathogens are expelled during coughing, sneezing, or talking and are transferred through the air to a host's mucous membranes, typically within 6 feet (2 m) of the infected person. In some circumstances, pathogens considered to be transmitted by droplets may also be transmitted by way of contact or airborne methods. For example, the common cold viruses are traditionally considered to be droplet-transmitted viruses, but the virus can also be transmitted by contact with fomites or by airborne microdroplets (according to some sources).

Airborne transmission occurs when microdroplets carrying a pathogen are generated by an infected person. Airborne transmission can also occur following coughing, sneezing, or talking. The novel severe acute respiratory syndrome coronavirus 2 (SARS-CoV-2), which causes an infection called coronavirus disease 2019 (COVID-19) leading to the COVID-19 pandemic, has been shown to spread through airborne transmission. Singing has recently been implicated in the airborne spread of the SARS-CoV-2 virus because it causes the generation and spread of aerosolized particles. The CDC has identified a wide variety of procedures performed in health care settings, known as aerosol-generating procedures (AGPs), which produce the much smaller microdroplets and require additional levels of personal protective equipment (PPE), including respirators. AGPs include suctioning of the airway, endotracheal intubation, nebulized medication administration, noninvasive ventilation, and other common medical procedures. These microdroplets are not stopped by traditional surgical or procedural masks, and they are known to remain suspended in the air for longer periods of time and travel great distances. Although airborne pathogens pass through the air and infect another host via the respiratory tract, these pathogens do not always cause respiratory illnesses. For example, chickenpox can be transmitted through the air (as well as through contact with mucous membranes) but does not cause a respiratory illness. The most well-known airborne-transmitted disease is tuberculosis (TB), which does affect the respiratory system as well as other organ systems.

> **CAUTION**
>
> ■ Hepatitis B virus (HBV) can survive for at least 1 week in dried blood on environmental surfaces or contaminated instruments, according to the CDC.
> ■ Vacuum cleaners are prohibited from the cleaning of broken glass under the Aerosol Transmissible Disease Standard (California Code of Regulations, Title 8, Section 5199).

Hierarchy of Controls

Both OSHA and the CDC conclude that preventing pathogen exposures requires a comprehensive program of strategies. A hierarchy of controls can be used to determine the most and least effective strategies **FIGURE 2-1**:

- Elimination: Physically remove the hazard.
- Substitution: Replace the hazard with a safe/safer alternative.
- Engineering controls: Isolate people from the hazard (eg, needleless devices, plastic capillary tubes, protective barriers).
- Administrative controls: Change the way people work (eg, providing vaccinations and promoting infection prevention and control training programs). This includes **work practice controls** (eg, hand hygiene, no needle recapping).
- PPE

In many occupational settings, it may be impossible to eliminate or replace an exposure hazard. If administrative, engineering, and work practice controls do not completely eliminate the risk of exposure, PPE, such as gloves, gowns, and eye protection, should be used.

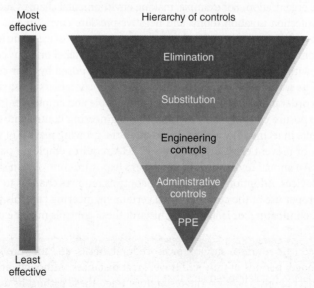

FIGURE 2-1 Hierarchy of controls.
© Jones & Bartlett Learning.

Administrative Controls

Administrative controls are policies and programs that manage and support the infection prevention program. Managerial and employee cooperation and adherence to the guidelines determine the effectiveness of these policies and programs. Examples of these controls include encouraging ill health care workers to stay home, infection prevention and control training programs, and vaccination programs. Vaccination programs are an integral part of disease prevention. Most health care workers have frequent contact with patients who have vaccine-preventable diseases, such as chickenpox or hepatitis B virus (HBV).

Most administrative controls seek to address the last chain in the chain of transmission: the susceptible host. Several factors influence susceptibility, including sex, race, age, genetics, comorbidities, and vaccination status, among others. Although factors such as sex and race cannot be altered, the employee can and should learn to reduce susceptibility by improving nutritional intake, reducing stress, exercising, and refraining from risky behaviors, in addition to maintaining current vaccinations. Several vaccines, including the one for HBV, are offered by employers free of charge to help employees stay protected from vaccine-preventable pathogens.

Activities such as disease or pathogen monitoring or surveillance can be grouped under the category of administrative controls. It is often necessary to change work practices as the prevalence of a particular disease or pathogen changes over time. Mitigation strategies such as limiting hospital visitation or proactively screening incoming patients can become effective administration controls in the midst of a local or widespread disease outbreak. Administrative controls within health care facilities can be isolation signs on patient rooms to warn staff and visitors that additional PPE or other precautions are required.

Engineering Controls

Engineering controls include any object that comes between you and the potential infectious material. Hand-washing facilities, eye stations, sharps containers close to the injection location, biohazard labels, self-sheathing needles or syringes, and needleless intravenous (IV) systems all are examples of engineering controls. A variety of protective devices are available to protect health care personnel while initiating IV access or administering injectable medications **FIGURE 2-2**. Engineering controls also include any effort to design safety into the tools and workspace organization. For example, making environmental changes such as adding air filtration systems, airborne infection isolation rooms and negative-pressure environments, air curtains, exhaust fans in patient transport vehicles, and other related systems to protect against exposure to airborne pathogens.

Regulated waste containers must be labeled with the biohazard label or color coded to warn people who may have contact with the containers of the potential hazard posed by their contents. Even if your facility considers all of its waste to be regulated waste, the waste containers must still bear the required label or color coding in order to protect new employees and people and employees from outside facilities.

Your employer's exposure control plan describes the engineering controls in use at your worksite. Significant improvements in technology are most evident in the growing market of safer medical devices that minimize, control, or prevent exposure incidents. OSHA requires employee participation in the selection of new devices. An annual review of your employer's exposure control plan should include identification of new safety devices. Adoption of engineering controls requires changes to your employer's plan and retraining in the proper use of the control. When certain engineering controls will reduce employee exposure by removing, eliminating, or isolating the hazard, these controls must be used.

CAL/OSHA

Cal/OSHA's regulation requires that hospitals, physicians, and other health care providers switch to safe needle systems.

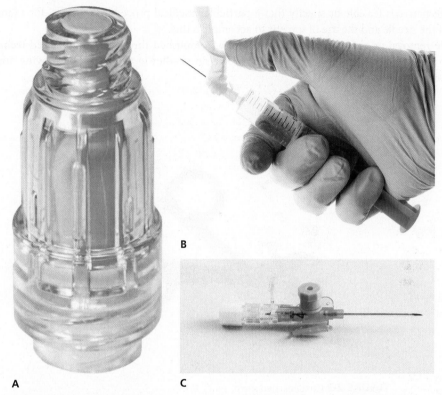

FIGURE 2-2 Protective intravenous (IV) devices. **A.** Needleless connector. **B.** Safety needle.
C. Retractable IV catheter.
A. Used with permission of Becton Dickinson International, Branch of Becton, Dickinson B.V; **B.** © ollo/iStock/Getty Images Plus/Getty Images;
C. © Frank Bienewald/Contributor/LightRocket/Getty Images.

Your employer is responsible for the full cost of instituting engineering and work practice controls. Your employer is also responsible for regularly examining, repairing, and/or replacing engineering controls as often as necessary to ensure that each control is maintained and that it provides the protection intended. Regularly scheduled inspections are required to confirm, for instance, that engineering controls, such as safety devices, continue to function effectively, that protective shields have not been removed or broken, and that physical, mechanical, or replacement-dependent controls are functioning as intended. Your employer may assign this task to you.

Contaminated Sharps

OSHA defines contaminated sharps as any contaminated object that can penetrate the skin, including, but not limited to, needles, scalpels, broken capillary tubes, and exposed ends of dental wires **FIGURE 2-3**.

Contaminated needles or other contaminated sharps must not be bent, recapped, or removed unless no alternative is feasible or such action is required by a specific medical procedure.

If a procedure requires shearing or breaking of needles, this procedure must be specified in the company's exposure control plan. An acceptable means of demonstrating that no alternative to bending, recapping, or removing contaminated needles is feasible or that such action is required by a specific medical procedure would be a written justification (supported by reliable evidence). This also needs to be included as part of the exposure control plan. The justification must state the basis for the determination that no alternative is feasible or specify that a particular medical procedure requires, for example, the bending of the needle and the use of forceps to accomplish this.

Needle removal or recapping needles must be accomplished through a one-handed technique or the use of a mechanical device. Do not attempt to recap needles in the back of a moving ambulance **SKILL DRILL 2-1**.

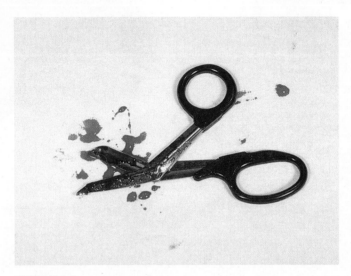

FIGURE 2-3 Contaminated sharp.
© Jones & Bartlett Learning. Courtesy of MIEMSS.

SKILL DRILL 2-1

One-Handed Recapping Technique

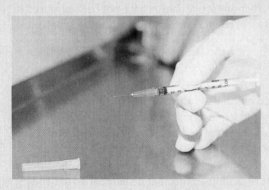

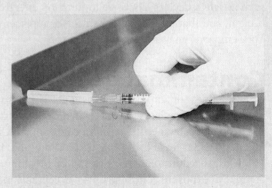

STEP 1 Using one hand, gently slide the needle into the needle cover.

STEP 2 Using the wall as support, apply gentle pressure to secure the needle cover.

© Jones & Bartlett Learning. Courtesy of MIEMSS.

Nurses (registered nurses and licensed practical nurses) sustain more needlestick injuries than any other type of health care worker in the United States, with 53% of all needlestick injuries. Non-health care providers working in health care fields, such as environmental services and laundry workers, sustain 25% of needlestick injuries. An overwhelming majority of the injuries were caused by needles that did not have a safe design. The needles were not shielded, recessed, or retractable. Most injuries occur during disposal of sharp devices. The CDC estimates that more than one-half of sharps injuries can be prevented by using safer devices. Despite a wide variety of administrative and engineering controls, there are approximately 600,000 needlestick injuries to US health care workers each year.

Reusable Sharps

Reusable sharps must be placed in clearly labeled, puncture-resistant, leak-proof containers immediately or as soon as possible after use until they can be reprocessed. The containers for reusable sharps are not required to be closable because it is anticipated that containers used for collecting and holding reusable sharps will be reused.

Reusable sharps, including pointed scissors that have been contaminated, must be decontaminated before reuse. Before cleaning, store the sharps in a container with a wide opening, and encourage people to use care in removing items.

For items to be considered properly cleaned and decontaminated, all visible blood or OPIMs must be rinsed off. Large amounts of organic debris interfere with the efficacy of the disinfecting and sterilization process. Consider using an enzymatic spray and closed container to keep blood and OPIM moist if there is going to be a delay in cleaning a used, contaminated item.

Use a mechanical means (forceps or tongs) to remove contaminated sharps from containers. Never reach into any container containing contaminated sharps with your hands. For example, employees must not reach into sinks filled with soapy water into which sharp instruments have been placed. Appropriate controls in such a circumstance would include the use of strainer-type baskets to hold the instruments and forceps to remove and immerse the items **FIGURE 2-4**.

When it is necessary to examine the contents of a container, pour the contents of the container out onto a surface for inspection. An example is inspecting a bag for illegal drugs that might contain a contaminated needle or syringe. (Wearing eye protection, disposable gloves, and a mask during this process is highly encouraged.) The intent is to provide conditions in which the contents can be seen and safely handled.

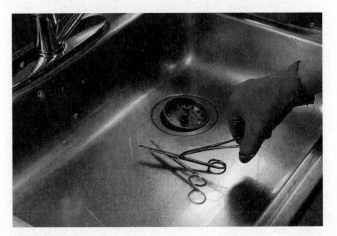

FIGURE 2-4 Use forceps to remove sharp objects from a container.
© Jones & Bartlett Learning.

Acceptable Sharps Containers

The Food and Drug Administration regulates sharps disposal containers as class II medical devices. OS-HA's Bloodborne Pathogens Standard establishes minimum design performance elements for sharps disposal containers. According to the Standard, a sharps container must meet four criteria to be considered acceptable. It must be closable, puncture-resistant, leak proof on sides and bottom, and labeled or color coded in accordance with the Standard **FIGURE 2-5**.

A sharps container may be made of a variety of products, including cardboard or plastic, as long as the four criteria are met. Duct tape may be used to secure a sharps container lid, but it is not acceptable if the tape serves as the lid itself.

A sharps container must have a warning label affixed to it. The Standard requires that warning labels "be affixed to containers of regulated waste, refrigerators, and freezers containing blood or other potentially infectious material; and other containers used to store, transport, or ship blood or other potentially infectious materials."

Using Sharps Containers

Contaminated sharps must be discarded immediately or as soon as feasible into an acceptable sharps container. Sharps containers must be easily accessible to personnel and located as close as possible to the immediate area where sharps are used or can be reasonably anticipated to be found. Sharps containers mounted onto walls should be 52 to 56 inches (132 to 142 cm) from the floor.

Sharps containers must be maintained upright throughout use, routinely replaced, and not overfilled.

The replacement schedule must be clearly outlined in the exposure control plan. When contaminated sharps are being moved from the area of use, the container must be closed immediately before removal or replacement to prevent spillage or protrusion of contents during handling, storage, transport, or shipping.

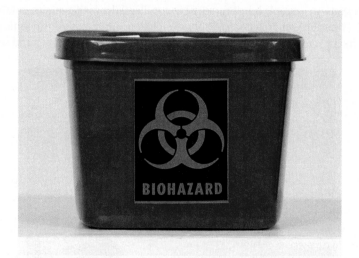

FIGURE 2-5 Biohazard symbols must be fluorescent orange or orange-red with letters or symbols in a contrasting color. These are attached to any container that is used to store or transport potentially infectious materials.
© American Academy of Orthopaedic Surgeons.

If leakage is possible or if the outside of the container has become contaminated, the sharps container must be placed in a secondary container that is closable and constructed to contain all contents and prevent leakage during handling, storage, transport, or shipping.

In areas such as correctional facilities, psychiatric units, or pediatric units, personnel may have difficulty placing sharps containers in the immediate use area. If workers in these units use a mobile cart to hold the sharps container, the sharps container should be locked to the cart.

Laundry facilities that handle contaminated laundry must have sharps containers easily accessible because of the incidence of needles mixed with laundry.

Facilities that handle shipments of waste that may contain contaminated sharps must also have sharps containers easily accessible in the event a package accidentally opens and releases sharps. All containers must be appropriately labeled with the name and address of the container's owner.

The Standard requires that reusable containers (such as those used to transport contaminated sharps for cleaning) not be opened, emptied, or cleaned manually or in any other manner that would expose employees to the risk of percutaneous injury. Remember that whatever goes into a *disposable* sharps container stays in the sharps container. At no time is anyone allowed to remove anything from a disposable sharps container. In many states, significant fines exist for anyone who removes or attempts to remove items from a disposable sharps container.

The Needlestick Safety Prevention Act

The Needlestick Safety Prevention Act became effective April 2001 and requires employers to:

- Implement new developments in control technology.
- Solicit nonmanagerial employees with direct patient care who are exposed to these potential hazards for input in the identification, evaluation, and selection of engineering and work practice controls.
- Maintain a log of percutaneous injuries from contaminated sharps.

Specific procedures for obtaining employee input might include informal problem-solving groups, employee participation in safety audits, workplace inspection, device evaluation, device pilot testing, and membership on a committee that consistently meets to review and audit reports of these activities.

Work Practice Controls

Work practice controls are the behaviors necessary to use engineering controls effectively. These include, but are not limited to, using sharps containers, using an eyewash station, implementing respiratory hygiene/cough etiquette, and washing your hands after removing PPE. An example of a work practice control is to immediately place contaminated sharps and PPE into the appropriate containers **FIGURE 2-6**.

All procedures involving blood or OPIMs must be performed in a manner that minimizes or eliminates splashing, spraying, splattering, and generation of droplets of these substances. This decreases the chances of direct exposure through spraying or splashing of infectious materials onto you and reduces contamination of surfaces in the general work area. Work practice controls must be regularly evaluated and updated to ensure their effectiveness.

Your employer must evaluate existing engineering and work practice controls and assess the feasibility of implementing new safety technology yearly. Many new products are introduced each year, not all of which may be appropriate for your work environment. These products should be evaluated with input from nonmanagerial employees whose responsibilities involve potential exposure to blood or OPIM. The specific process for evaluating safety technology is not outlined by the Standard; however, experience has shown that a productive review process might include the following steps:

1. Form a multidisciplinary team that follows a timetable for completing timely evaluations.

2. Identify priority areas and give the highest priority assessment to any work area or practice in which percutaneous injuries have occurred. Emphasize safety devices with features that will have the greatest effect on preventing occupational injury.

3. Conduct the evaluation with participants who will actually use the selected device.

Hand Hygiene and Handwashing Facilities

Handwashing is one of the most effective methods of preventing transmission of pathogens. It is required that you wash your hands after removal of gloves and other PPE **FIGURE 2-7**.

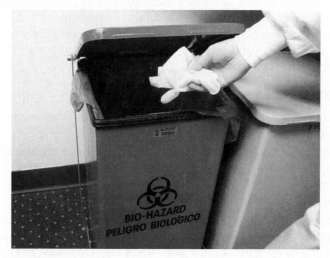

FIGURE 2-6 Properly dispose of protective equipment in biohazard containers.
Courtesy of Kimberly Smith and Christine Ford/CDC.

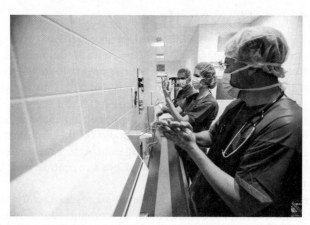

FIGURE 2-7 Handwashing is a primary means of preventing transmission of bloodborne pathogens.
© wavebreakmedia/Shutterstock.

Employers are required to provide handwashing facilities that are readily accessible to all employees. The Standard specifies that the handwashing facilities must be situated so that you do not have to use stairs, doorways, and corridors, which might result in environmental surface contamination.

When the provision of handwashing facilities is not feasible (such as in an ambulance or police vehicle), the employer must provide either an appropriate antiseptic hand cleanser (eg, alcohol foam) or antiseptic towelettes. Alcohol-based hand cleaners must contain at least 60% ethanol. Be aware of products that contain methanol, which can be harmful or fatal when ingested by people drinking it as an alcoholic beverage substitute. Waterless and alcohol-based hand sanitizers do not remove gross contamination, many chemicals, and other harmful substances. If you use antiseptic hand cleansers or towelettes, you must wash your hands (or other affected area) with soap and warm water as soon as possible after contact with blood or OPIMs **FIGURE 2-8**. Certain pathogens such as *Clostridioides difficile* are not susceptible to alcohol-based cleaners so handwashing with soap and water is essential when treating infectious patients with those conditions.

Respiratory Hygiene/Cough Etiquette

Combining the strategies of respiratory hygiene/cough etiquette helps minimize the transmission of aerosol-transmissible pathogens in health care settings. These strategies include:

- Covering the mouth and/or nose during coughing and sneezing and using tissues or masks to contain respiratory secretions.
- Disposing of tissues and/or masks contaminated with respiratory secretions.
- Ensuring hand hygiene (eg, handwashing with alcohol-based hand sanitizer, soap and water, antiseptic hand wash or wipes) after contact with respiratory secretions and contaminated objects or materials.
- Ensuring spatial separation of at least 6 feet (2 m) from others when coughing.
- Providing tissues and no-touch receptacles.
- Providing alcohol-based hand sanitizer dispensers.
- Ensuring that handwashing supplies are available at sink locations.

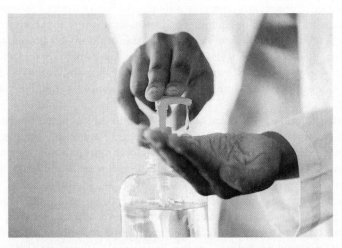

FIGURE 2-8 Use a waterless handwashing solution if there is no running water available. Be sure to wash your hands with soap and running water as soon as possible.
© SDI Productions/Getty Images.

Cleaning Work Surfaces

The term work area indicates an area in which work involving exposure or potential exposure to blood or OPIMs exists, along with the potential contamination of surfaces.

The term *worksite* not only refers to permanent fixed facilities, such as hospitals, dental and medical offices, or clinics, but also covers temporary nonfixed workplaces. Examples of such facilities include, but are not limited to, ambulances, bloodmobiles, temporary blood collection centers, and any other non-fixed worksites that have a reasonable possibility of becoming contaminated with blood or OPIMs. Your employer will identify which work surfaces require inspection for contamination with blood or OPIMs and regularly scheduled decontamination. These surfaces could include, but are not limited to, exam tables, counters, floors, ambulance interiors, police vehicles, and wastebaskets.

A regular inspection and cleaning schedule should be followed. The schedule must consider location (exam room versus patient waiting area), type of surface (carpet versus hard floor), type of soil present (gross contamination versus minor splattering), and procedure and tasks performed (laboratory analysis versus patient care). The cleaning schedule must occur at least weekly or after completion of tasks or procedures, after contamination of surfaces, or at the end of a shift if there is a possibility of contamination. Cleaning in patient care areas and public spaces may range in complexity from frequent wipe-downs of high-touch surfaces (doorknobs, armrests, countertops, etc) to a full terminal clean of every item and surface in a given area.

Do not use your hands to clean up any broken glass that may be contaminated. Instead, use a dustpan and brush, cardboard, or tongs **SKILL DRILL 2-2**. The tools used in cleanup (such as forceps) must be properly decontaminated or discarded after use. Contaminated broken glass must be placed in a bio-hazard sharps container. Placing broken glass in a plastic bag may put others at risk for an occupational exposure incident. You must be given specific information and training with respect to this task.

Eating; drinking; smoking; applying cosmetics, lotions, or lip balm; and handling contact lenses are prohibited in work areas where there is a reasonable likelihood of occupational exposure to blood or OPIMs.

Personal Protective Equipment

When the potential for exposure exists despite engineering and work practice controls, employers must provide PPE. PPE is used to protect you from contamination of skin or mucous membranes and puncture wounds. PPE is specialized clothing or equipment that you wear or use for protection against hazards. It includes equipment such as nitrile or vinyl gloves, washable or disposable gowns, aprons, face shields, masks, eye protection, fluid-resistant leg and shoe coverings, laboratory coats, cardiopulmonary resuscitation (CPR) microshields, and resuscitation bags. PPE prevents blood or OPIMs from contacting or passing through to your work or street clothes, undergarments, skin, eyes, mouth, or other mucous membranes **FIGURE 2-9**.

Laboratory coats and uniforms that are used as PPE must be laundered by the employer and not sent home with the employee for cleaning. Although many employees have traditionally provided and laundered their own uniforms or laboratory coats, the employer must provide, clean, repair, replace, and/or dispose of the item if it is used as PPE. The biohazard symbol must be affixed to any biohazard waste or contaminated materials, such as PPE laundry.

Your employer is responsible for providing PPE at no expense to you. PPE must be provided in appropriate sizes and placed within easy reach for all employees. Your employer must evaluate the job task as well as the type and associated risk of exposure expected and, based on the determination, select the appropriate personal protective clothing. For example, laboratory coats or gowns with long sleeves must be used for procedures in which exposure of the forearm to blood or OPIMs is reasonably anticipated to occur.

SKILL DRILL 2-2

Cleaning a Contaminated Spill

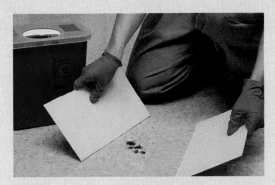

STEP 1 When cleaning up broken glass, wear gloves and/or other PPE.

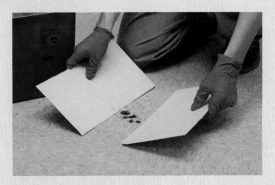

STEP 2 Do not clean up broken glass with your hands. Instead, use a dustpan and brush, cardboard (as shown), or tongs.

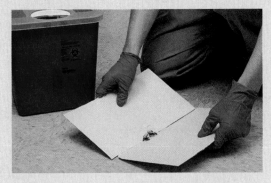

STEP 3 Slide pieces of cardboard under broken glass.

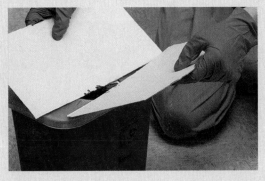

STEP 4 Place broken glass in an appropriate sharps container. Do not place in a plastic bag. Placing broken glass in a plastic bag may put others at risk for exposure.

© Jones & Bartlett Learning.

It is necessary for you to be trained in the proper use of PPE. Report to your supervisor when any equipment is not available (such as a missing protective shield) or not in working order (such as a hole in an apron).

If blood or OPIMs contaminate your clothing, you must remove the clothing as soon as feasible and place it in an appropriately designated area or container.

Resuscitator devices must be readily available and accessible to employees who can reasonably be expected to perform resuscitation procedures. Emergency ventilation devices also fall under the scope of PPE and therefore must be provided by the employer for use in resuscitation. This includes masks, mouthpieces,

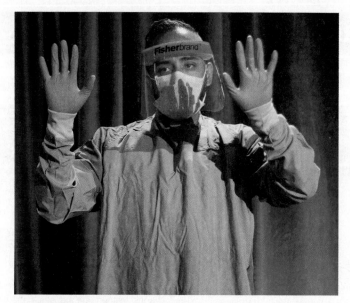

FIGURE 2-9 Full personal protective equipment includes gloves, gown, mask, and eye shield.
© David McNew/Stringer/Getty Images News/Getty Images.

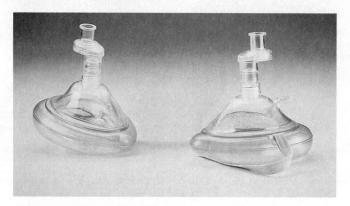

FIGURE 2-10 Barrier devices, such as a pocket mask, are necessary in providing artificial ventilations.
© American Academy of Orthopaedic Surgeons.

resuscitation bags, and shields and overlay barriers **FIGURE 2-10**. Consider using a mechanical compression device if CPR compressions must be performed on high-risk patients **FIGURE 2-11**. It may be difficult to keep complex PPE intact, or you might risk early exhaustion while wearing complex PPE and performing manual chest compressions. These would not technically be considered PPE; however, they provide a similar function of protecting workers performing resuscitation of patients with highly contagious pathogens.

Gloves

Gloves must be used when there is reasonable anticipation of employee hand contact with blood, OPIMs, mucous membranes, or nonintact skin; when performing vascular access procedures; or when handling or touching contaminated surfaces or items.

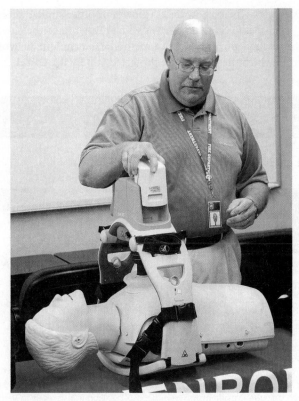

FIGURE 2-11 LUCAS chest compression device.
© ZUMA Press Inc/Alamy Stock Photo.

Gloves are not necessary when administering intramuscular or subcutaneous injections as long as bleeding that could result in contact with blood or OPIMs is not anticipated. Gloves are not necessary when blood or OPIMs are not present or do not have the possibility of occurring.

It is important to consider that the use of gloves is required for any situation that might reasonably be anticipated to result in an exposure to blood or OPIMs. For example, the use of pneumatic tube systems for the transport of laboratory specimens requires that all employees should regard the contents as hazardous and must wear gloves when removing specimens from the tube system carrier.

FYI

- Studies have shown that gloves provide a barrier, but that neither vinyl, latex, nor nitrile disposable gloves are completely impermeable.
- Disinfecting agents may cause deterioration of the glove material. Washing with surfactants could result in wicking or enhanced penetration of liquids into the glove via undetected pores, thereby transporting blood and OPIMs into contact with the hand. For this reason, disposable (single-use) gloves may not be washed and reused. In many areas, facilities are replacing their disposable latex gloves with single-use nitrile gloves due to increased sensitivity to latex in the general population. In addition, nitrile offers some protection against chemicals, such as those used for disinfection of equipment.

Hypoallergenic gloves, glove liners, powderless gloves, or other similar alternatives must be readily available and accessible at no cost to those employees who are allergic to the gloves normally provided.

Removing used latex or vinyl gloves requires a methodical technique to avoid contaminating yourself with the materials from which the gloves have protected you **SKILL DRILL 2-3**.

SKILL DRILL 2-3

Proper Glove Removal Technique

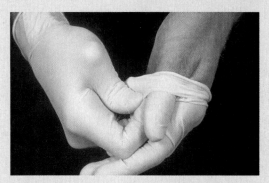

STEP 1 Begin by partially removing one glove. With your other gloved hand, pinch the first glove at the wrist—being certain to touch only the outside of the first glove—and start to roll it back off your hand, inside out. Leave the exterior of the fingers on that first glove exposed.

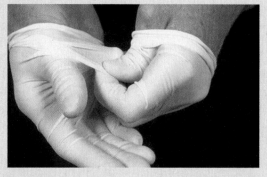

STEP 2 Use the still-gloved fingers of the first hand to pinch the wrist of the second glove and begin to pull it off, rolling it inside out toward the fingertips as you did with the first glove.

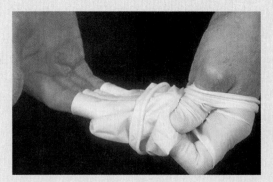

STEP 3 Continue pulling the second glove off until you can pull the second hand free.

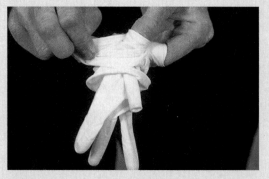

STEP 4 With your now-ungloved second hand, grasp the exposed inside of the first glove and pull it free of your first hand and over the now-loose second glove. Be sure that you touch only clean, interior surfaces with your ungloved hand. Dispose of gloves in a biohazard container or a sealed plastic bag. Then, wash your hands with soap and running water.

Latex Allergy

Natural rubber latex (NRL) is a glove material that has been used in the health care environment for barrier protection for many years. In response to reported NRL allergy in some patients and health care workers, measures have been recommended to reduce the risk of NRL allergy in workers.

The signs and symptoms of latex allergies include rashes, inflammation (immediate or delayed), respiratory irritation, asthma, and, in rare cases, shock. The groups that fall in the high-risk category for latex allergies include health care workers and workers in the latex industry. The occupational issues with latex allergies include more than just the affected employee. Workers with latex sensitivities must use nonlatex gloves, and their coworkers must use either nonpowdered latex or nonlatex gloves. It is common for individuals with spina bifida, a birth defect involving the spinal column, or frequent exposure to repeated surgical procedures early in life to develop sensitivities to NRL.

Gowns and Leg/Shoe Coverings

A gown may be necessary while interacting with some patients. A gown provides additional protection from large amounts of blood or OPIMs. Situations where a gown may be required include childbirth or interaction with patients who have experienced major trauma. Gowns are also included in the guidelines for implementing contact precautions. Fluid-resistant or barrier leg coverings and shoe coverings should be used when large volumes of blood or OPIMs might be encountered, or where personnel must transition in and out of areas where infectious agents, requiring droplet or contact precautions, are present.

Eye Protection and Face Shields

Eye protection can minimize mucous membrane exposure to bloodborne pathogens or OPIMs. Reasonably anticipated spattering or generation of droplets would also necessitate the use of eye protection and a mask or face shield to prevent contamination of the mucous membranes of the eyes, nose, and mouth. Whenever you need to wear a face mask as PPE, you must also wear eye protection.

In addition, some forms of eye protection will prevent the wearer from foreign body objects entering the eyes. If you are wearing your personal glasses, you must use side shields and plan to decontaminate your glasses and side shields according to the schedule determined by your employer. Even with side shields, regular prescription glasses do not provide full splash protection. People who wear prescription glasses will need to have safety glasses that go over them or have prescription safety glasses made. If the employer cannot provide glasses or a face shield to cover the employee's glasses safely, the employer is required to purchase specialty prescription glasses at no cost to the employee.

> **CAUTION**
>
> Whenever clothing is soaked with blood or OPIMs, the employee must be permitted to change into fresh garments before continuing with work. A paramedic on an emergency call whose garments become soaked with blood or OPIMs but who continues to the next call without a change of clothing would be in violation of the Standard.

Respirators and Masks

Surgical and procedural masks are physical barriers that provide protection from large splashes of blood or OPIMs. They can be worn by health care workers to limit contamination of patient wounds or work areas, such as during surgery. Placing a surgical or procedural mask on an infected patient can minimize the spread of respiratory secretions, trapping large particles during exhalation, talking, coughing, or sneezing. Surgical masks are not designed to prevent inhalation of smaller airborne contaminants and do not qualify as respirators.

Respirator masks are used to reduce occupational exposure to smaller airborne contaminants, including aerosolized particles typically defined as being ≤5 micrometers (µm) in length. Respirators work by removing contaminants, such as microdroplets that contain bacteria or viruses, from the air. Diseases that can be transmitted by aerosolized particles requiring health care and other personnel to wear respirators include TB and COVID-19. All employees required to wear a respirator must have a medical evaluation and training and be fit-tested for their specific respirator model at no cost to the employee.

Standard and Transmission-Based Precautions

The CDC has outlined categorized precautions for employees to implement to reduce or eliminate the transmission of pathogens. These precautions incorporate elements of engineering controls, work practice controls, and PPE.

Some patients will require not only the use of standard precautions but also transmission-based precautions depending on the route of transmission of the particular pathogen with which the patient is infected. Transmission-based precautions encompass three subsets: contact, droplet, and airborne precautions.

Standard Precautions

Standard precautions refer to an aggressive, standardized approach to infection control. This group of infection prevention practices applies to all patients (and animals in research settings), regardless of suspected or confirmed diagnosis or presumed infection status. According to the concept of standard precautions, treat all bodily substances as if they contain pathogens, regardless of the perceived risk of the source.

Standard precautions are a combination and expansion of what have been known in the past as *universal precautions* and *body substance isolation*. As such, standard precautions include recommendations for hand hygiene, respiratory hygiene/cough etiquette, environmental controls, safe injection practices, cleaning and disinfecting, and the use of gloves, gown, mask, eye protection, or face shield as needed TABLE 2-1.

TABLE 2-1 Standard Precautions for the Care of All Patients in All Health Care Settings

Standard Precautions
1. Ensuring hand hygiene before and after patient contact and when touching potentially contaminated materials (regardless of whether gloves are worn)
2. Donning personal protective equipment (PPE) to include gloves, gown, surgical/procedural mask, respirators, and eye and face protection depending on anticipated health care worker–patient interaction
3. Ensuring safe injection practices
4. Ensuring respiratory hygiene/cough etiquette
5. Donning a surgical/procedural mask or respirator for insertion of catheters or injection of material into spinal and/or epidural spaces (eg, myelogram, spinal or epidural anesthesia)
6. Donning surgical/procedural mask, respirator, and/or eye protection to protect mucous membranes (eyes, nose, and mouth) during procedures and patient care activities that may produce potentially infectious splashes or sprays
7. Handling or transporting patient care equipment soiled with potentially infectious material to designated area in appropriate container according to facility policies that prevent secondary transmission
8. Routinely following facility's policies for environmental and high-touch surface cleaning and disinfection in between patients

9. Handling, processing, and transporting used linen that has been soiled with potentially infectious materials in a manner that prevents secondary transmission
10. Following occupational health and bloodborne pathogens requirements to reduce the risk of infection from contaminated equipment and inherently risky patient care procedures

Transmission-Based Precautions (Combined With Standard Precautions)

Contact Precautions—Used in prevention of pathogens transmission by direct or indirect contact with patients or environmental items. Additionally applied in the presence of fecal incontinence, vomiting, wound drainage, or other potentially infectious material discharges:

1. Place the patient in a private room. Facility protocols may allow for cohorting of individuals with the same type of infection.
2. Don PPE before entering the patient's room and discard before exiting.
3. Ensure spatial separation of at least 3 feet (1 m).
4. Ensure hand hygiene.
5. Wear gloves.
6. Wear a gown.
7. Limit patient transport. When transport is necessary, place a surgical mask (if tolerated) on the patient and encourage the patient to practice respiratory hygiene/cough etiquette.
8. Dedicate patient care equipment to one patient whenever possible. If common use of equipment among patients is unavoidable, clean and disinfect equipment before use on another patient.
9. Apply additional requirements specifically for preventing the spread of carbapenem-resistant pathogens.

Droplet Precautions—Used in prevention of pathogens transmission by close respiratory or mucous membrane contact with respiratory secretions:

1. Place the patient in a private or cohort room.
2. Don surgical mask, eye protection, and face shield when within 6 feet (2 m) of the patient.
3. Ensure spatial separation of at least 6 feet (2 m) between patients (curtain separation if possible).
4. Limit patient transport. When transport is necessary, place a surgical mask (if tolerated) on the patient and encourage the patient to practice respiratory hygiene/cough etiquette.
5. If possible, nonimmune health care workers should not care for patients with vaccine-preventable, droplet-transmissible diseases (eg, varicella, mumps, influenza type A and B). This will likely include the coronavirus disease 2019 (COVID-19) vaccine as it becomes widely available to health care providers.

Airborne Precautions—Used in prevention of airborne pathogens transmission (eg, tuberculosis [TB], severe acute respiratory syndrome [SARS], and measles):

1. Place the patient in an airborne infection isolation room, previously known as a negative-pressure room.
2. Ensure respiratory protection, including N95 or higher respirator (disease-specific recommendations).
3. Limit patient transport. When transport is necessary, place a surgical mask (if tolerated) on the patient and encourage the patient to practice respiratory hygiene/cough etiquette.
4. If possible, nonimmune health care workers should not care for patients with vaccine-preventable airborne diseases (eg, measles, chickenpox, and influenza).
5. Apply additional guidelines for specific prevention of TB.

Data from Centers for Disease Control and Prevention, 2007.

Substances Requiring Standard Precautions

Standard precautions apply to the following substances:

- Blood
- Saliva
- Mucus

- Sweat
- Semen
- Vaginal secretions
- Cerebrospinal fluid
- Synovial fluid
- Pleural fluid
- Any body fluid with visible blood
- Any unidentifiable body fluid

Transmission-Based Precautions

Transmission-based precautions are recommended to provide additional precautions beyond standard precautions to interrupt the transmission of pathogens. Transmission-based precautions can be used for patients with known or suspected pathogens that can be transmitted by air, droplets, or contact. These precautions should be used *in addition to* standard precautions.

Contact Precautions

Contact precautions are used for infections spread by skin-to-skin contact or contact with other surfaces (eg, linen, countertops, doorknobs), such as methicillin-resistant *Staphylococcus aureus* and *C. difficile*.

Droplet Precautions

Droplet precautions are used for infections spread in large droplets by coughing, talking, or sneezing, such as influenza.

Airborne Precautions

Airborne precautions are used for infections that spread small particles in the air, such as TB and COVID-19. They include hand hygiene, eye protection or face shield, gloves, gown, dedicated patient care items, private or cohort rooms, limited patient movement and/or transport, airborne isolation rooms, and respiratory protection, including an N95 or higher respirator mask.

The OSHA Bloodborne Pathogens and Respiratory Protection Standards have greatly improved employee safety through training and prevention measures. They have also influenced manufacturers to introduce new engineering controls (such as needleless systems) and produce a wide variety of products that create a safer work environment and provide greater personal protection. Despite these advances, pathogens continue to pose a significant occupational health risk for employees. Continued implementation of these Standards remains an essential component to maintaining a safe working environment.

FYI

Although success in eliminating the causes of serious illness and disease is mixed, bioterrorism is the newest challenge. Terrorists may attempt to infect entire communities with deadly diseases or toxins. Many of these biologic agents are found in nature and can be manufactured to increase their effectiveness. In addition, the ease of international travel makes it more likely that any biologic agent purposely released into the general public could spread around the world in a matter of hours or days. Preparedness activities must be initiated at all levels and sectors. Hospitals must prepare for and practice steps necessary to diagnose, treat, and rapidly isolate potential victims of a biologic terrorist attack.

The foundational information concerning pathogens also applies to bioterrorism agents. Prevention strategies, such as standard and transmission-based precautions, can be used to mitigate some of the effects of these agents. For additional information regarding bioterrorism, visit http://emergency.cdc.gov/bioterrorism/.

Site-Specific Work Page

Employee Training

1. Labeling methods at this worksite include the following:

   Color: _____

   Biohazard symbol (label): _____

   Words: _____

   Red bag: _____

2. The person to notify if I discover regulated waste containers, refrigerators containing blood or OPIMs, or contaminated equipment without proper labels is: _____

   _____

3. At my worksite, we are expected to adhere to standard and transmission-based precautions:
   - ❏ Yes
   - ❏ No

4. According to my employer's exposure control plan, sharps containers are to be inspected

   every _____ and replaced when _____.

5. Three examples of engineering controls at my worksite are:

   _____

   _____

   _____

   _____

   _____

6. The handwashing station nearest to my worksite is located at:

   _____

   _____

PREP KIT

Vital Vocabulary

decontamination The use of physical or chemical means to remove, inactivate, or destroy bloodborne pathogens on a surface or item to the point where they are no longer capable of transmitting infectious particles and the surface or item is rendered safe for handling, use, or disposal.

fomites Inanimate objects, such as desks, faucets, or doorknobs, that have been contaminated with pathogens.

hand hygiene A general term that applies to any one of the following: (1) handwashing with plain (nonantimicrobial) soap and water; (2) antiseptic handwash (soap containing antiseptic agents and water); (3) antiseptic hand rub (waterless antiseptic product, most often alcohol-based, rubbed on all hand surfaces); or (4) surgical hand antisepsis (antiseptic hand wash or antiseptic hand sanitizer performed preoperatively by surgical personnel to eliminate transient hand flora and reduce resident hand flora).

handwashing facilities These include alcohol sanitizer dispensers, sinks with soap and hand-drying supplies, or other Centers for Disease Control and Prevention-approved facilities.

needleless systems Devices that do not utilize needles for (1) the withdrawal of body fluids after initial venous or arterial access is established, (2) the administration of medication or fluids, and (3) any other procedure involving the potential for occupational exposure to bloodborne pathogens due to percutaneous injuries from contaminated sharps.

pandemic A disease outbreak that spreads across multiple countries or continents.

respiratory hygiene/cough etiquette A combination of measures designed to minimize the transmission of respiratory pathogens via droplet or airborne routes in health care settings.

severe acute respiratory syndrome coronavirus 2 (SARS-CoV-2) The virus that causes an infection called coronavirus disease 2019 (COVID-19), which primarily affects the lungs and can lead to respiratory failure and death.

source individual Any individual, living or dead, whose blood or other potentially infectious materials may be a source of occupational exposure to the employee. Examples include, but are not limited to, hospital and clinic patients; clients in institutions for the developmentally disabled; trauma patients; clients of drug and alcohol treatment facilities; residents of hospices and nursing homes; human remains; and people who donate or sell blood or blood components.

terminal clean An intense disinfecting process occurring at least every 24 hours to kill pathogens and remove organic material from the environment in order to make it safe to use again by other patients, visitors, and health care providers.

transmission-based precautions Recommended to provide additional precautions beyond standard precautions to interrupt transmission of pathogens; these include airborne precautions, droplet precautions, and contact precautions.

vaccine A suspension of inactive or killed microorganisms administered orally or injected into a human to induce active immunity to infectious disease.

PREP KIT continued

vector An animal or insect (eg, fleas, mosquitoes, birds, rodents) that transmits pathogens, such as rabies, malaria, or West Nile virus, to human hosts.

work area The area where work involving risk of exposure or potential exposure to blood or other potentially infectious materials exists, along with the potential contamination of surfaces.

Check Your Knowledge

1. A gown that frequently rips or falls apart under normal use would be considered appropriate PPE.

   A. True

   B. False

2. The exposure control plan describes the engineering controls in use at a worksite.

   A. True

   B. False

3. Duct tape may be used to secure a sharps container lid.

   A. True

   B. False

4. When cleaning up potentially contaminated broken glass, you may use a dustpan and brush, cardboard, or an industrial vacuum cleaner.

   A. True

   B. False

5. You may launder your own PPE, but only if this is clearly specified in the exposure control plan.

   A. True

   B. False

6. Gloves must be used where there is reasonable anticipation of contact with blood or OPIMs to employee hands.

   A. True

   B. False

7. Your employer must supply hypoallergenic gloves at no cost to employees who are allergic to the gloves normally provided.

   A. True

   B. False

8. Containers of contaminated laundry do not need to be labeled.

   A. True

   B. False

9. Handwashing is not required after the removal of gloves.

   A. True

   B. False

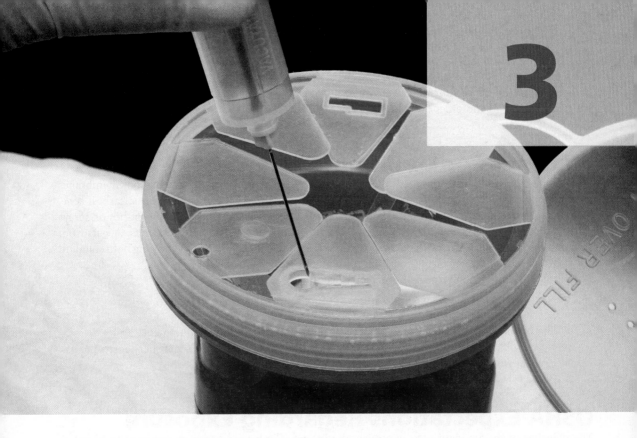

3

Bloodborne Pathogens

Overview

The Occupational Safety and Health Administration (OSHA) Bloodborne Pathogens Standard applies to all pathogenic microorganisms spread by exposure to infected blood or other potentially infectious materials (OPIMs) from human or occupational animal sources. It is not feasible to address all possible pathogens, so this chapter will focus on hepatitis B virus (HBV), hepatitis C virus (HCV), human immunodeficiency virus (HIV), and Ebola virus disease (EVD). Information about other pathogens may be added into your training by your employer based on your geographic location and job description.

What Are Bloodborne Pathogens?

Bloodborne pathogens are disease-causing microorganisms, such as viruses, bacteria, or parasites, that are carried in blood and other body fluids. They may be transmitted by direct or indirect exposure to blood or OPIMs.

Transmission of Bloodborne Pathogens

Bloodborne pathogens are transmitted when blood or OPIMs come in contact with mucous membranes or nonintact skin. Nonintact skin includes, but is not limited to, cuts, abrasions, burns, rashes, acne, paper cuts, and hangnails. Bloodborne pathogens may also be transmitted by blood splashes or sprays (direct contact), contaminated items or surfaces (indirect contact), or punctures, wounds, or cuts from contaminated sharps. Contact with blood or OPIMs should be avoided **FIGURE 3-1**. Using both standard and contact precautions enhances protection from bloodborne pathogens.

Transmission of bloodborne pathogens may occur via:

- Mother to infant (through the placenta, exposure during birth, or breast milk)
- Sexual contact with an infected person (oral, vaginal, or anal)
- Sharing of contaminated needles, syringes, or other intravenous drug equipment
- Needlesticks (up to 30% chance of infection) or penetrating injuries by other sharp instruments
- Contact with contaminated items or surfaces
- Blood splashes or sprays

OSHA Expectations Regarding Exposure

The objective of the Standard is to minimize or eliminate the hazard posed by exposure to blood or OPIMs; however, occupational exposure to a bloodborne pathogen may occur.

If you are exposed to bloodborne pathogens, a confidential medical evaluation is to be made immediately available to you, the injured employee. The word *immediately* is used in the Standard to emphasize the importance of prompt medical evaluation and prophylaxis. An exact time frame cannot be stated because the effectiveness of postexposure prophylactic measures varies depending on the infecting organism.

Medical evaluation must be confidential and protect your identity and test results. You and your employer should expect that current Centers for Disease Control and Prevention (CDC) guidelines will be used to guide postexposure prophylaxis and treatment. It is the employer's responsibility to ensure

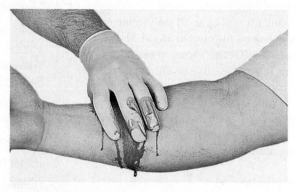

FIGURE 3-1 Always wear gloves to prevent contamination. Wearing two pairs of gloves may be helpful in some instances.
© American Academy of Orthopaedic Surgeons.

that your medical records are kept confidential. Your records cannot be disclosed without your express written consent to any person within or outside the workplace, except as required by law. Your employer will have a copy of the health care provider's written description of the incident.

Reporting Requirements

What Is an Occupational Exposure Incident?

An occupational exposure incident occurs if you are in a work situation and come in contact with blood or an OPIM.

For OSHA record-keeping purposes, an occupational bloodborne pathogens exposure incident (eg, a needlestick, laceration, or splash) is classified as an injury because it is usually the result of an instantaneous event or exposure **FIGURE 3-2**.

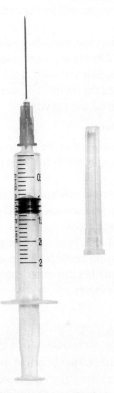

FIGURE 3-2 An uncapped needle can cause an injury.
© Iana Alter/Shutterstock.

For OSHA record-keeping purposes, the Log of Work-Related Injuries and Illnesses (Form 300) is used to note the extent and severity of each case. Any employee who has had an occupational exposure to blood or OPIM will not have their name entered on the OSHA 300 log. Other fields on the 300 form may be filled in as long as they do not specifically identify the injured employee.

Reporting an Incident

The goal of reporting an incident is to ensure that an employee receives timely access to medical services and to identify and adopt other methods or devices to prevent exposure incidents from recurring.

> **FYI**
>
> Employers do not have a specific right to know the actual results of the source individual's blood testing, but they must ensure that the information is provided to the evaluating health care professional.

The employee must report the incident to their supervisor within the prescribed time frame. OSHA requires that the following information be reported:

- Date and time of the exposure incident
- Job classification of the exposed employee
- Worksite location where the exposure incident occurred
- Work practices being followed
- Engineering controls in use at the time, including a description of the device in use (such as the type and brand of sharp involved in the exposure incident)
- Protective equipment or clothing that was used at the time of the exposure incident
- Procedure being performed when the incident occurred
- The exposed employee's training for the activity

Cal/OSHA also requires the following:

- Identification of the body part involved in the exposure incident
- Documentation of the engineering controls in use at the time if the sharp had engineered sharps injury protection
- Description of whether the protective mechanism was activated and whether the injury occurred before the protective mechanism was activated, during activation of the mechanism, or after activation of the mechanism, if applicable
- If the sharp had no engineered sharps injury protection, the injured employee's opinion as to whether and how such a mechanism could have prevented the injury
- The employee's opinion about whether any other engineering, administrative, or work practice control could have prevented the injury

> **CAL/OSHA**
>
> Cal/OSHA requires a sharps injury log that records the date and time of each sharps injury resulting in an exposure incident, as well as the type, brand, and model (if indicated) of the device involved in the exposure incident.

> **OSHA**
>
> OSHA does not require redrawing of the source individual's blood specifically for HBV, HCV, and HIV testing without the consent of the source individual.

After an incident has been reported, your employer will need to identify and document the source individual and obtain consent and make arrangements to have the source individual tested as soon as possible to determine HIV, HCV, and HBV infection. It should be documented when legally required consent to test the blood is not obtained.

It may not always be feasible to identify the source individual. Examples of when you may be unable to identify the source individual include needlesticks caused by unmarked syringes left in laundry or those involving blood samples that are not properly labeled, as well as incidents occurring where state or local laws prohibit such identification.

> **FYI**
>
> State laws may vary. Please check with your instructor regarding testing and test result confidentiality laws in your state.

> **OSHA**
>
> As part of bloodborne pathogens training, OSHA requires that information be provided to employees on the appropriate actions to take and people to contact in an emergency involving blood or OPIMs.

Your blood may be tested for HBV, HCV, and/or HIV only with your consent. OSHA encourages employees to consent to blood collection at the time of exposure. The results of HIV testing must be made in person and cannot be given over the telephone or by mail. Even if you choose not to undergo testing, counseling and evaluation of reported illnesses are available to you.

You may choose to have your blood drawn but not tested, and stored for 90 days. The 90-day time frame gives the employee the opportunity to obtain knowledge about baseline serologic testing after exposure incidents and to participate in further discussion, education, or counseling. If you elect not to have the blood tested, the sample will be disposed of after 90 days.

Hepatitis Viruses

Hepatitis means inflammation of the liver. Hepatitis has a variety of causes, including drugs, poisons, toxins, and bloodborne pathogens. Viral hepatitis is the leading cause of liver cancer and the need for liver transplants in the United States. This section will focus on two viral causes of hepatitis encountered in occupational settings: HBV and HCV. With an effective HBV vaccine available for many years,

HBV affects far fewer individuals than HCV. HBV infects approximately 21,200 people annually in the United States, with between 800,000 and 900,000 estimated chronic infections. It is currently estimated by the CDC that approximately 2.4 million people are living with chronic HCV in the United States, with roughly 50,000 new cases reported each year.

There is also a hepatitis D virus (HDV) that exists primarily outside the United States; however, the individual must have a concurrent infection with HBV for HDV to be transmitted successfully. Two additional hepatitis viruses, hepatitis A virus and hepatitis E virus, are typically spread by contaminated foods or drinks and are not discussed further in this text.

FYI

- If you have an exposure incident to another person's blood or an OPIM, immediately wash the exposed area with warm water and soap.
- If the exposed area was in your mouth, rinse your mouth with water immediately.
- If the exposure was in your eyes, flush with clean water, sterile eye irrigating solution, or normal saline (if available). Irrigate from the nose side of the eye toward the outside to avoid flushing the blood or OPIM into the other eye. A quick rinse will likely be inadequate; you want to irrigate the area completely with water.
- Your employer will have site-specific work practices to follow in the event of an emergency.

Hepatitis B Virus

Hepatitis B remains a concern for health care workers and many related occupations that might be exposed to blood or OPIM. The incidence of HBV has declined due to the widespread use of the HBV vaccine and other prevention measures though the incidence in the United States has remained relatively constant over the past decade. People at higher risk for HBV than the general population include infants of mothers with HBV, those who engage in risky behaviors (eg, drug abuse, sexual promiscuity), and those who have preexisting health conditions, such as another liver condition or HIV. The HBV can remain live and potentially infectious on surfaces for up to 7 days.

Clinical Presentation

The incubation period (time between exposure and development of signs and symptoms) is between 45 and 160 days. Signs and symptoms of HBV may include:

- Jaundice (yellow appearance of the skin or whites of the eyes)
- Malaise (fatigue)
- Fever
- Loss of appetite
- Nausea and vomiting
- Abdominal pain
- Dark urine
- Gray-colored stools
- Joint pain
- Elevated liver function tests

According to the CDC, approximately 95% of adult HBV cases resolve without further complication; however, about 5% of individuals with new infections will become asymptomatic carriers or progress to chronic hepatitis infection, which causes significant injury to the liver over time. The rates of chronic infection are much higher when infants and young children are infected early in life.

FYI

- **Immunization** with hepatitis B vaccine should be made available within 10 working days of initial assignment to the job.
- Your employer cannot require you to use your health insurance or your family insurance to pay for the cost of the vaccine.
- To learn more about CDC recommendations, visit http://www.cdc.gov/hai.

FYI

- Advances in the field of antiviral therapy and the use of protease inhibitors might change the recommendations for treatment and follow-up for HCV and HIV infection; therefore, it is important to work closely with your health care professional and use current CDC guidelines.
- All antiviral drugs have been associated with significant side effects. Protease inhibitors may interact with other medications and cause serious side effects.

Treatment

HBV is best addressed through supportive care, which means signs and symptoms are addressed as they appear. In some cases, antiviral medications may be beneficial. For chronic HBV, liver transplantation may be indicated. There is no cure for infection with HBV.

Postexposure Treatment

Provide immediate care to the exposure site as follows:

- Wash the affected area with soap and water.
- If applicable, flush mucous membranes with copious amounts of running water.

All decisions about postexposure prophylaxis are made in consultation with your health care professional. In some cases, hepatitis B immunoglobulin (prescribed medication containing antibodies to the virus) and hepatitis B vaccination may be indicated, if the person has not already been vaccinated. Postexposure treatment for HBV should begin within 24 hours and no later than 7 days after exposure.

Prevention and Control

Standard and contact precautions, along with work controls, reduce the incidence of exposure and are key tools in preventing the spread of HBV in the occupational setting. If an exposure does occur, vaccination is the best protection against contracting HBV. The CDC reports that, for an unvaccinated person, the risk of contracting HBV from a single needlestick or a cut exposure to HBV-infected blood ranges from 6% to 30%. For a vaccinated person who has developed immunity to HBV, there is virtually no risk for contracting HBV from occupational exposure.

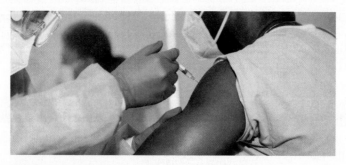

FIGURE 3-3 Vaccination against hepatitis B is possible.
© Mongkolchon Akesin/Shutterstock.

Vaccination

The hepatitis B vaccine has been available since 1982 and does not contain any live components. The vaccine is given in a series of three shots over a 6-month period **FIGURE 3-3**. The first shot is given within 10 working days of the initial assignment. The second shot is given 1 month later, and the third shot is given 5 months after the second dose. Immunity following HBV vaccine is highest in infants at 95%; however, it declines to approximately 75% when the vaccine is administered to individuals older than 60 years. For current information regarding the side effects and contraindications of the vaccination, consult your health care professional or request to see the information insert provided in the vaccination package. Women who are pregnant or breastfeeding should inform their primary medical practitioner before receiving any vaccination.

All employees, including temporary, part-time, and volunteer workers, with routine occupational exposure to blood or OPIMs have the right to receive the injection series against HBV at no personal expense. The Standard requires that your employer offer the vaccine to you at a convenient time and place during normal work hours. If travel away from the worksite is necessary to obtain vaccination, your employer is responsible for the transportation costs.

OSHA's intent is to have your employer eliminate obstacles to your acceptance of the vaccine; however, the term *made available* emphasizes that you may refuse the series by signing the hepatitis B vaccine declination form (see Appendix B). If you change your mind while still covered under the Standard at a later date, you may still receive the vaccine at no cost. Refer to your employer's guidelines regarding the declination or refusal to receive the HBV vaccine.

If your job requires ongoing contact with patients or blood and you are at ongoing risk for injuries with sharp instruments or needles, the CDC recommends that you be tested for antibodies to the HBV surface antigen (HBsAg) 1 to 2 months after the completion of the three-dose vaccination series. If you do not respond to the primary vaccination series by producing adequate amounts of antibodies, you may choose to be revaccinated with a second three-dose vaccine series and then retested for HBsAg. Nonresponders should be medically evaluated to rule out immune dysfunction.

Hepatitis C Virus

Hepatitis C is the most common chronic bloodborne infection in the United States. It is not as easily transmitted following a needlestick as HBV; however, as indicated earlier, there is a far greater incidence of HCV in the general population. No vaccine exists for HCV, making it a greater risk of transmission following occupational exposure.

Transfusion-associated cases occurred before blood donor screening and are now extremely rare. Injectable drug abuse has accounted for a substantial proportion of HCV infections in the United States.

Other people at high risk for HCV include infants of mothers with HCV, those who engage in risky behaviors (eg, drug abuse, unprotected sex), those who share personal care items that may have blood on them (eg, razors and toothbrushes), and those who have preexisting health conditions, such as another liver condition or HIV.

> **CAUTION**
>
> Infection with one form of hepatitis does not prevent infection with another form of hepatitis. For example, a person with an HCV infection may still become infected with HBV.

Clinical Presentation

The incubation period for HCV is between 14 and 180 days. Signs and symptoms of HCV mimic those of HBV, although up to 75% of people with acute HCV exhibit no signs and symptoms. Even without any symptoms, carriers can still transmit the virus to others. Between 5% and 25% of acute HCV cases result in chronic liver disease. In the United States, HCV is the major cause of liver damage requiring liver transplantation.

Treatment

HCV is best addressed through supportive care, just like HBV. Antiviral medications may have some benefit in the early stages of the disease and may be used as a treatment option for chronic infection. Liver transplantation is also a treatment option when liver damage is severe.

Postexposure Treatment

Provide immediate care to the exposure site as follows:

- Wash the affected area with soap and water.
- If applicable, flush mucous membranes with copious amounts of running water.

> **FYI**
>
> - HCV has specifically been included wherever HIV and HBV are mentioned in the regulation.
> - A recent meta-analysis revealed that health care workers were infected with HCV at rates significantly statistically higher than the general population; however, personal risk factors could not be evaluated due to study limitations.
> - Needlestick injury is the only occupational risk factor that has been associated with HCV infection.
> - Referral to a specialist in liver disease may be necessary to properly manage an HCV infection.
> - In follow-up studies of health care workers who sustained percutaneous exposures to blood from HCV-positive patients, the incidence of HCV conversion averages between 2% and 10%.

Based on the CDC guidelines from July 2020, no postexposure prophylaxis (prevention of infection) is recommended. Guidelines indicate periodic testing to monitor if HCV infection occurs. All decisions about postexposure laboratory testing and treatment interventions should be made in consultation with your health care professional. The baseline test for HCV and liver function tests should occur as soon as possible after exposure and should be repeated 3 to 6 weeks, then again 4 to 6 months after the exposure. There are a variety of potentially curative medication options available following occupational exposure to HCV. Direct-acting antiviral medications represent new powerful treatment options not previously available. The treatment regimen following HCV exposure depends on a wide variety of factors including the genotype of the virus strain and the patient's response to the initial viral infection. However, there are medication options for infection after occupational exposure.

Prevention and Control

Standard and contact precautions, along with work controls, reduce the incidence of exposure and are key tools in preventing the spread of HCV in the occupational setting. A hepatitis C vaccination does not currently exist.

Human Immunodeficiency Virus

HIV leads to acquired immunodeficiency syndrome (AIDS). This syndrome describes a condition in which the body is unable to fight off infection or destroy mutated cells, thus leaving it vulnerable to opportunistic infections and cancer.

The CDC estimates that there are more than 1.2 million people living with HIV in the United States **FIGURE 3-4**. HIV is undiagnosed in approximately 14% (1 in 7) of those people and they are unaware

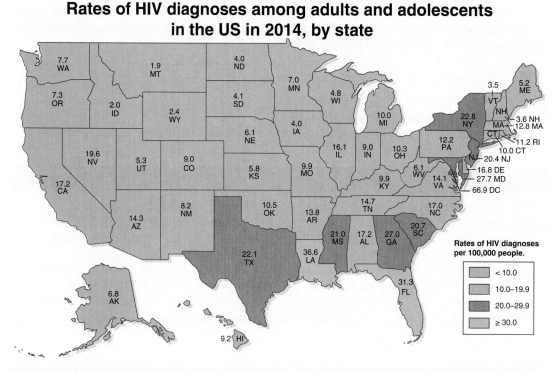

FIGURE 3-4 Estimated number of people living with human immunodeficiency virus and/or acquired immunodeficiency syndrome in 2014.

Courtesy of Centers for Disease Control and Prevention. Data from CDC. Diagnoses of HIV infection in the United States and dependent areas, 2014. HIV Surveillance Report 2015;26.

of their infection. Current HIV infection rates are approximately 38,000 people per year in the United States. Since the beginning of the epidemic in 1981, an estimated 700,000 people with AIDS have died in the United States.

Routes of Transmission

People at higher risk for HIV infection than the general population include infants of mothers with HIV, those who engage in risky behaviors (eg, drug abuse, unprotected sexual encounters), and those with preexisting health conditions that affect the immune system (eg, malnourishment, another systemic disease) who also have potential exposure to HIV. Occupational transmission of HIV most frequently occurs from puncture injuries from contaminated sharps; however, there have been a few documented transmissions through nonintact skin and mucous membranes. One worker became HIV positive after a splash of HIV-contaminated blood to the eyes. Even with these documented cases, seroconversion (development of HIV antibodies) is rare, occurring only 3 times out of every 1,000 exposures to HIV (0.3%).

Incubation Period

The period between exposure to HIV and detectable antibodies in the blood is approximately 1 month. The incubation period may be 1 to 15 years or more for a confirmed HIV infection to develop into AIDS. Many people who are infected with HIV experience no symptoms during this latency period. AIDS diagnosis occurs when the patient tests positive for HIV, has a CD4 count less than 200, or certain opportunistic infections develop. The CD4 count measures T-helper lymphocytes (CD4 cells), a type of white blood cells that are essential components of the immune system. Common opportunistic infections in the patient with HIV include tuberculosis, pneumocystis pneumonia, candidiasis (thrush), and herpes simplex virus.

Clinical Presentation

The common symptoms of acute HIV infection are similar to the flu and may include night sweats, headache, fever, fatigue, swollen lymph nodes, and muscle or joint pain. Absolute determination of HIV infection can only be established by testing.

Currently, no cure or vaccine exists for HIV or AIDS. With combinations of certain antiretroviral treatment medications, a person's HIV viral load may decrease to nondetectable levels on serum blood tests. This treatment regimen will greatly reduce the risk of transmitting the virus to others. Individuals in high-risk situations or engaged in high-risk behaviors might be prescribed a combination medication for "preexposure prophylaxis (PrEP)" as a preventive measure. According to the CDC, PrEP reduces the infection rate following sexual intercourse by 99% and following intravenous drug use by 74% when taken as prescribed.

FYI

The CDC reports that the risk of infection after a needlestick or a cut exposure to HIV-infected blood is approximately 0.3%.

Treatment

People with confirmed HIV seroconversion may be given antiretroviral medications to slow the progression of the disease. Supportive care addresses other health issues as they arise.

Postexposure Treatment

Provide immediate care to the exposure site as follows:

■ Wash the affected area with soap and water.
■ If applicable, flush mucous membranes with copious amounts of running water.

Postexposure prophylaxis of HIV may include antiretroviral medications. There is no cure for infection with HIV. All decisions about postexposure prophylaxis should be made in consultation with your health care professional. Current guidelines do not recommend postexposure prophylaxis for all occupational bloodborne exposures. If treatment with antiviral medications or other medications is recommended, treatment should begin within 72 hours of postexposure.

Prevention and Control

There is currently no vaccination for HIV.

Standard and contact precautions, along with work controls, reduce incidence of exposure and are key tools in preventing the spread of HIV in the occupational setting.

Ebola Virus Disease

EVD, formerly known as Ebola hemorrhagic fever, is a viral infection that has had numerous outbreaks in West Africa, with infected individuals spreading the disease into other parts of the world including the United States. This highly contagious and infectious virus has a fatality rate ranging from 40% to 90% depending on the particular outbreak and origin site. Outbreaks occur after a human acquires the virus from an infected animal and begins passing it to others. Once the outbreak begins, it passes easily from person to person, making it difficult to contain. There are reports of accidental EVD infections resulting from laboratory mishaps and lingering concern that EVD will be used as a bioterrorism agent.

Routes of Transmission

EVD spreads easily from person to person through direct contact and fomite transmission. The virus is present in the blood, urine, saliva, sweat, feces, vomit, and other body fluids of infected individuals. Health care workers and close contacts of infected patients are most at risk. Transmission is only possible when the infected person is experiencing symptoms of the disease.

Incubation Period

EVD symptoms typically begin 6 to 12 days following exposure; however, they may develop as late as 21 days after exposure.

Susceptibility

Two versions of EVD vaccine are currently available. One received Food and Drug Administration (FDA) approval in 2019. The other is still being used on a research protocol at the time of this writing.

Clinical Presentation

Symptoms of EVD are as follows:

- Fever
- Headache
- Muscle and joint pain
- Abdominal pain
- Weakness and fatigue
- Diarrhea and vomiting (severe)
- Unexplained hemorrhaging, bleeding, or bruising

Postexposure Treatment

The treatment of EVD is supportive. These patients often require vast amounts of intravenous fluids and electrolytes to offset the massive fluid volume losses through vomiting and diarrhea. Significant hemorrhage may require blood product administration to correct anemia or coagulopathy. Persistent hypotension (low blood pressure) may require vasopressor medications. Critical patients may require supplemental oxygen or endotracheal intubation. Two antiviral medications for the treatment of severe EVD were approved by the FDA in late 2020.

Prevention and Control

Health care and related workers who come into contact with individuals who have known or suspected EVD should be meticulous with personal protective equipment (PPE) use while interacting with these individuals. Any unnecessary procedures, including blood draws, that create additional risk of exposure should be avoided. Use disposable medical and patient care equipment whenever possible. Any rooms or vehicles that are used for patients with EVD should have a full terminal clean, with environmental services workers in adequate PPE in place. PPE should include protection for the face and eyes; fluid-resistant gowns; impervious leg and shoe coverings; and durable, fluid-resistant gloves. Wearing two pairs of gloves may be helpful in some instances. EVD transmission has occurred during removal of PPE (doffing), so a careful process and use of an assistant is recommended.

Site-Specific Work Page

Employee Training

In addition to HBV, HBC, and HIV, the instructor also reviewed the following bloodborne pathogens:

Pathogen: _____

Prevention and control: _____

Clinical features and disease history: _____

Postexposure prophylaxis and follow-up: _____

Pathogen: _____

Prevention and control: _____

Clinical features and disease history: _____

Postexposure prophylaxis and follow-up: _____

Pathogen: _____

Prevention and control: _____

Clinical features and disease history: _____

Postexposure prophylaxis and follow-up: _____

The required medical records are maintained by _____at (location)

_____

Medical records are kept for the duration of my employment plus 30 years: ❏ Yes   ❏ No

Medical care at my worksite is provided by: _____

Medical records are provided to me or to anyone having written consent from me within 15 days:
❏ True   ❏ False

The person responsible for evaluating if an exposure incident meets OSHA record-keeping requirements is:

_____

Hepatitis B vaccine is provided by _____at (location)

_____

The health care professional's written opinion concerning hepatitis B immunization is limited to whether the employee requires the vaccine and whether the vaccine was administered: ❏ True   ❏ False

My question about HBV is: _____

My question about HCV is: _____

My question about HIV is: _____

My question about another bloodborne pathogen is: _____

PREP KIT

Vital Vocabulary

acquired immunodeficiency syndrome (AIDS) A collection of signs and symptoms that results from human immunodeficiency virus.

antibodies Specialized immunity proteins that bind to an antigen to make it more visible to the immune system.

antigen A substance that causes antibody formation.

Ebola virus disease (EVD) A viral infection that causes profound body fluid loss, hemorrhage, and is frequently fatal. This virus typically originates in West Africa but has the ability for widespread transmission as people travel.

hepatitis Inflammation of the liver.

hepatitis B virus (HBV) A virus that causes liver infection. It ranges in severity from a mild illness lasting a few weeks (acute) to a serious long-term (chronic) illness that can lead to liver disease or liver cancer.

hepatitis C virus (HCV) A virus that causes liver infection. HCV infection sometimes results in an acute illness but most often becomes a chronic condition that can lead to cirrhosis of the liver and liver cancer.

human immunodeficiency virus (HIV) A virus that infects immune system blood cells in humans and renders them less effective in preventing disease.

immunity Resistance to an infectious disease.

immunization A process or procedure by which resistance to an infectious disease is produced in a person.

jaundice A yellowing of the skin associated with hepatitis infection.

opportunistic infections Illnesses caused by various organisms, many of which often do not cause disease in people with healthy immune systems.

percutaneous Occurring through the skin, such as drawing blood with a needle.

prophylaxis Protective measures designed to prevent the spread of disease.

Check Your Knowledge

1. For which virus is there an effective vaccine?

   A. HIV

   B. HCV

   C. HBV

2. If you do not respond to the first hepatitis B immunization series, you may be revaccinated with a second series.

   A. True

   B. False

3. List two symptoms of hepatitis.

4. Symptoms are not specific in the diagnosis of HIV infection.

   A. True

   B. False

5. HIV is the virus that causes AIDS.

   A. True

   B. False

PREP KIT continued

6. Postexposure treatment of HIV and HCV is controversial and should be discussed with a physician immediately after exposure.

   A. True

   B. False

7. It is necessary to report as much detail as possible about an exposure incident.

   A. True

   B. False

8. Hepatitis B vaccine is offered at no cost to you.

   A. True

   B. False

9. It is possible to diagnose infection with HIV, HBV, and HCV with a blood test.

   A. True

   B. False

10. Occupational exposure occurs primarily through needlestick injuries.

    A. True

    B. False

11. Which virus poses the greatest risk for infection after a puncture injury?

    A. HBV or HCV

    B. HIV

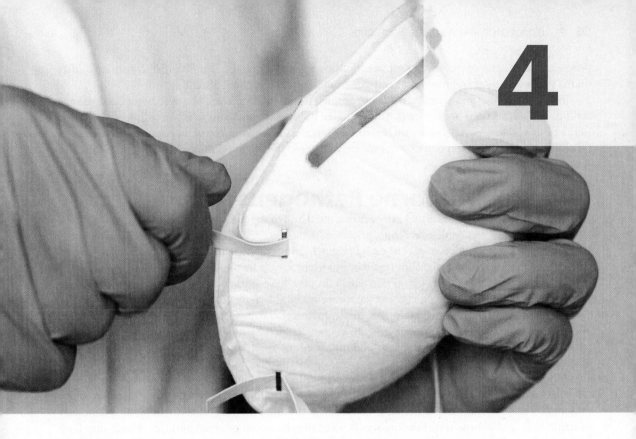

4

Airborne Pathogens

Overview

The outbreak of coronavirus disease 2019 (COVID-19), the disease caused by the severe acute respiratory syndrome coronavirus 2 (SARS-CoV-2) virus, in early 2020 demonstrates how quickly an illness can affect countries all around the world in a very short time. In travelers without evidence of illness on departure, symptoms developed soon after arrival at their destinations. In some cases, these travelers unknowingly spread the infection to friends, family, and health care workers. A small number of individual travelers were later identified as key spreaders of COVID-19 early in the pandemic.

Stopping the spread of infectious diseases requires high levels of suspicion and strong local, national, and international cooperation to mount a quick response to the sudden appearance of any unusual infectious disease. Air travel has allowed people to reach places all over the world. As more and more people travel, the risk of spreading serious infectious diseases increases. It is essential to keep up to date on the various diseases and how to remain safe from the spread of these diseases.

This chapter describes several airborne or droplet-spread pathogens encountered in the occupational setting. The descriptions are not exhaustive but give basic facts about the airborne pathogens common in the United States. A brief discussion regarding a few worldwide airborne pathogens is also included in this chapter. Information on other pathogens may be found in the appendices.

What Are Airborne Pathogens?

Airborne pathogens are diseases that can be transmitted by droplet or airborne/aerosolized routes. Droplets are generated when people talk, cough, or sneeze. Although droplet transmission is technically a contact route, it is placed in its own special category due to its propensity to travel over short distances and directly into the respiratory tract. However, it is important to note that it is possible to become infected by contact routes, such as touching fomites on which droplets have landed. An example would be touching a table with infected droplets and rubbing your eyes or nose, thereby providing a portal of entry for the disease-causing pathogen. Prevention strategies for droplet transmission include respiratory hygiene/cough etiquette, visual alerts, personal protective equipment (PPE), hand hygiene, masking of the source patient (infected patient) during transport, and separate rooms or cohorting (placing patients with the same disease in a room together).

Much smaller aerosolized particles are also released during coughing, talking, singing, and sneezing. Aerosolized particles are also released during aerosol-generating procedures, such as endotracheal intubation, aerosol medication delivery, suctioning, cardiopulmonary resuscitation, or pulmonary function testing. Airborne transmission occurs when droplet nuclei or small particles (which may have been milled to smaller particles due to environmental factors, such as sneeze velocity, thermal effects, humidity, and wind) enter a susceptible host. Pathogens that are carried by the airborne route can be transported over long distances or air currents and require several preventive strategies. These strategies include those listed in the previous paragraph and the addition of ventilation systems, such as airborne infection isolation rooms (AIIRs).

COVID-19

Coronavirus disease 2019 (COVID-19) was first discovered in Wuhan, China, in December 2019, and in a short period of time caused a global pandemic. It is a respiratory virus caused by the SARS-CoV-2 virus. This particular virus is considered "novel" because it has never been previously isolated. It has many characteristics similar to the SARS and Middle East Respiratory Syndrome (MERS) virus outbreaks from 2003 and 2012, respectively. SARS, MERS, and COVID-19 viruses are in the coronavirus family. Much of the science regarding COVID-19 is still evolving as new research is conducted and new treatment strategies continue to be developed. According to the Centers for Disease Control and Prevention (CDC), these three viruses likely originated in bats. At the time of this book's printing, there were more than 297.2 million confirmed cases in the United States, with over 538,000 deaths and with new records being set frequently.

Route of Transmission

COVID-19 is primarily spread from person to person through droplet transmission **FIGURE 4-1**. Additional routes include much smaller aerosolized respiratory particles spread through contaminated objects and surfaces (fomites). The role of aerosol spread remains the subject of ongoing research, and it may eventually be determined to be the primary route of transmission of COVID-19. At the time

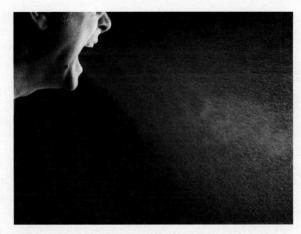

FIGURE 4-1 Coughing and sneezing create droplets and aerosols.
© James Klotz/Shutterstock.

of this book's printing, COVID-19 continues to have largely uncontrolled community spread despite ambitious public health efforts promoting face mask wearing, social distancing, and limits on large gatherings.

Susceptibility

COVID-19 is posing an enormous public health challenge. At the time of this book's printing, several vaccines against COVID-19 are being released to the general public as an emergency measure. Health care workers and minority groups appear to be infected with COVID-19 at rates well above the general population in the United States. COVID-19 tends to cause greater complications in older adults and those with serious underlying medical conditions such as diabetes, heart disease, and obesity. People infected with COVID-19 may be symptomatic or asymptomatic. In most people infected with the virus, signs and symptoms develop within 2 to 14 days. Those infected are most infectious to others days before any symptoms develop, which has undoubtedly contributed to widespread pandemic as people are infectious when they are not aware of their illness.

Clinical Presentation

- Fever or chills
- Cough
- Difficulty breathing
- Fatigue
- Muscle or body aches
- Headache
- New loss of taste or smell
- Sore throat
- Congestion or runny nose
- Nausea or vomiting
- Diarrhea

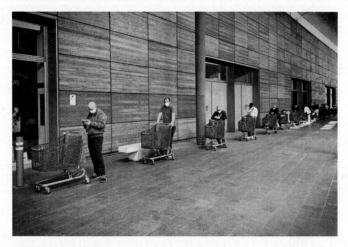

FIGURE 4-2 Social distancing line outside a grocery store during the COVID-19 pandemic.
© MikeDotta/Shutterstock.

Postexposure Treatment

Treatment of COVID-19 is generally supportive and is based on the severity of symptoms. Many patients require supplemental oxygen. Severe cases require prolonged endotracheal intubation and mechanical ventilation. Other supportive treatment strategies include the use of high-flow nasal oxygen and awake prone positioning (ie, placing the patient on their stomach for several hours each day). Several medications were tested early during the pandemic outbreak. At the time of this book's printing, the corticosteroid medication dexamethasone (Decadron) and the antiviral medication remdesivir (Veklury) and two monoclonal antibody medications casirivimab and imdevimab are the only promising medications in the management of COVID-19. A wide variety of other medications and treatment strategies are currently under evaluation. It is likely that additional treatment strategies will continue to emerge as more is learned about COVID-19.

Prevention and Control

A wide variety of public health initiatives are currently implemented to attempt to control the spread of COVID-19. In the United States, the three primary strategies are consistent wearing of face masks, creating a "social distance" of 6 feet between individuals in public areas, and avoiding large gatherings **FIGURE 4-2**. The implementation varies dramatically across the United States and around the globe. Currently, within the United States, these steps might be either completely voluntary or may be made mandatory by a formal public health order or an executive order from a governor. The prospect of long-term immunity following COVID-19 is currently unproven as antibodies to SARS-CoV-2 appear to diminish rapidly over time. Additionally, some reinfections have occurred and may be underreported. The science of COVID-19 continues to evolve.

Influenza (Seasonal)

Influenza, or flu, is a viral illness that is easily spread from person to person. It primarily affects the respiratory system. Flu epidemics occur in late fall to early spring. Flu infection rates are highest for children and people older than 65 years and anyone with health care conditions that increase their risk for complications.

Several types of influenza virus exist. Many share the same characteristics, with a few minor exceptions.

Route of Transmission

Seasonal influenza is primarily transmitted through droplets. When a person sneezes, the moisture from the airway moves forcefully and quickly through a narrow opening. If the moisture and droplets are large, they travel short distances and can be involved in direct person-to-person transmission. Influenza may also be transmitted from contaminated surfaces (fomites). According to the CDC, individuals may spread influenza to others 1 day *before* symptoms begin and can still spread it 5 to 7 days *after* the illness began.

Incubation Period

The incubation period is approximately 1 to 4 days.

Susceptibility

Anyone not rendered immune by vaccination is susceptible. Susceptibility is predicated on a variety of factors. One preventive measure both the employer and the employee can implement to reduce the incidence of illness due to influenza is yearly vaccinations. As with all vaccines, effectiveness will vary depending on age, disease, and immune status. The CDC has stated, "How well the flu vaccine works (or its ability to prevent flu illness) can range widely from season to season and can be affected by a number of factors, including characteristics of the person being vaccinated, the similarity between vaccine viruses and circulating viruses, and even which vaccine is used." Seasonal influenza vaccines are developed to match the anticipated virus strains that predominate in a given year. In many years, the influenza vaccines are effective at controlling seasonal influenza. Occasionally, the seasonal influenza vaccines are not effective against the predominant virus strains and cause a more severe influenza season. No vaccinations are 100% effective, so it is important to implement other preventive strategies, such as hand hygiene and respiratory hygiene/cough etiquette.

Clinical Presentation

Primary symptoms:

- Fever
- Malaise
- Muscle aches
- Body aches
- Sore throat
- Runny nose
- Cough

Other potential symptoms and complications:

- Diarrhea
- Eye infections
- Pneumonia
- Respiratory distress
- Other severe and potentially life-threatening complications

Postexposure Treatment

General postexposure management principles apply to all exposed people. Antiviral medications may be indicated for postexposure treatment.

Proper handwashing is the simplest yet most effective way to control disease transmission. The longer the germs remain with you, the greater their chance of getting through natural barriers (such as skin or mucous membranes). Although soap and water are not protective in all cases, in certain cases their use provides excellent protection against further transmission from your skin to others. If no running water is available, you should use waterless handwashing substitutes.

Prevention and Control

Standard and droplet precautions should be implemented for all suspected or confirmed cases. Vaccinate as recommended by a health care practitioner. Prescription antiviral drugs approved for influenza (based on seasonal outbreak data) may be of some benefit in treating most strains of flu infection in humans; however, influenza viruses can become resistant to these drugs, reducing their effectiveness. For these medications to be most effective, they must be taken within 48 hours of the first symptoms.

FYI

- Each year in the United States, the CDC estimates there are several thousand deaths due to the influenza virus. During the 2019-2020 influenza season, there were 22,000 related deaths in the United States.
- The collection of yearly viral cultures is critical because the virus isolated from the culture provides specific information about influenza strains and subtypes. This information is used to guide formulation of vaccines for the next flu season.

Influenza (Swine and Avian)

During 2009, a new strain of influenza of swine (pig) origin (H1N1) began to spread. Within a few months, the "swine flu" reached pandemic proportions and caused the United States to declare a public health emergency. Many similarities exist between the H1N1 strain and other types of influenza. Currently, prevention strategies include standard, contact, and airborne precautions, including the use of an N95 or higher respirator mask.

Avian influenza (H5N1) is caused by an influenza type A viral subset that normally occurs only in birds but has recently been found to cross over to humans. Symptoms are similar to those of seasonal influenza. Prevention includes avoiding contact with poultry and other birds suspected or known to be infected. Avoid eating uncooked or undercooked poultry or poultry products. If you are sick, stay at home, except to get medical attention. Cover your mouth and nose when you cough or sneeze.

Tuberculosis

Tuberculosis (TB) is a disease caused by the bacterium *Mycobacterium tuberculosis*. Approximately 80% to 85% of TB infections occur in the lungs, with the remaining cases occurring in nonpulmonary sites, such as the central nervous system, kidneys, lymph nodes, and skeletal system. TB is a serious and often a fatal disease if left untreated. The distribution of pulmonary versus nonpulmonary TB varies throughout the world. The CDC estimates that up to 13 million people in the United States have latent TB infections.

After infection with the TB bacterium, two TB-related conditions can occur: latent TB infection (LTBI) and active TB disease. In LTBI, bacteria can live inside the human host for years without causing any health effects. The only sign of LTBI is a positive reaction to the tuberculin skin test (TST) or TB blood test. People who have LTBI cannot spread the disease to others but their risk of the development of active TB disease is 5% to 10%.

Active TB disease occurs when the body's immune system cannot stop the bacteria from multiplying. People with active TB disease can spread the disease to others.

Route of Transmission

TB is a disease that primarily spreads from person to person through droplet nuclei suspended in the air by coughing, sneezing, or talking. Under normal circumstances, the mechanism for transmission used by *M. tuberculosis* is not very efficient. Infected air is easily diluted with uninfected air. *M. tuberculosis* is one of those germs that typically causes no illness in a new host. In fact, many patients with TB do not even transmit the infection to family members.

Incubation Period

The incubation period for *M. tuberculosis* ranges from 2 to 10 weeks. Those people who are immunocompromised may have a more rapid clinical deterioration, such as pediatric patients or those with human immunodeficiency virus (HIV).

Susceptibility

Anyone is susceptible to TB infection. People who are immunocompromised, are on long-term corticosteroid therapy, or have HIV are at higher risk of the development of active TB disease. Other medical risk factors for the development of TB are diabetes, gastrectomy (removal of the stomach), immunosuppressive therapy, or cancers and other malignancies.

Clinical Presentation

- Cough
- Production of sputum
- Weight loss
- Loss of appetite
- Weakness
- Fever
- Night sweats
- Malaise
- Chest pain
- Hemoptysis

Hemoptysis, the coughing up of blood, may also occur, but usually not until after a person has had active TB disease for some time.

Postexposure Treatment

If a TB infection is confirmed before you become ill, preventive therapy is almost 100% effective. The treatment for active TB disease is a long process. Most regimens take 6 to 9 months to complete. There is an intensive treatment phase lasting approximately 2 months, followed by a continuation phase lasting 4 to 7 months. There are 10 medications currently approved for TB. The CDC recommends using a combination of four different medications depending on your situation. The medications are isoniazid (INH), rifampin (Mycobutin), ethambutol (Myambutol), and pyrazinamide (Tebrazid).

There are other preferred treatment regimens for patients with latent TB, those with HIV, and those with medication-resistant TB. There are also other preferred treatment regimens for pregnant patients with TB and for children with TB.

Prevention and Control

The CDC recommends a combination of administrative, engineering, and PPE controls to minimize TB transmission. These strategies are used in combination to promote workplace safety and to provide the employee with maximum protection against occupational exposure to *M. tuberculosis*. Under these guidelines, the control of TB is to be accomplished through the early identification, isolation, and treatment of people with TB; the use of engineering and administrative procedures to reduce the risk of exposure; and the use of respiratory protection. Respiratory protection measures should include all elements of Occupational Safety and Health Administration (OSHA) 29 CFR 1910.134.

In order to ensure a safe working environment and to meet the OSHA General Duty Clause requirements, employers should provide the following:

1. An assessment of the risk for transmission of *M. tuberculosis* in the particular work setting.

2. A protocol for the early identification of people with active TB.

3. Training and information to ensure employee knowledge of the method of TB transmission, its signs and symptoms, medical surveillance and therapy, and site-specific protocols, including the purpose and proper use of controls. (Failure to provide respirator training is citable under OSHA's general industry standard on respirators.)

4. Medical screening, including preplacement evaluation, administration, and interpretation of TST or the T-cell interferon gamma release assay (T-IGRA) blood test.

5. Evaluation and management of workers with positive skin tests or a history of positive skin tests who are exhibiting symptoms of TB, including work restrictions for infectious employees.

6. Airborne infection isolation rooms for patients with suspected or confirmed infectious TB. These isolation rooms and areas in which high-hazard procedures are performed should be single-patient rooms with special ventilation characteristics that are properly installed, maintained, and evaluated to reduce the potential for airborne exposure to *M. tuberculosis*.

7. Institution of exposure controls specific to the workplace, which include the following:

   - Administrative controls are policies and procedures to reduce the risk of employee exposure to infectious sources of *M. tuberculosis*. An example is a protocol to ensure rapid detection of people who are likely to have an active case of TB.
   - Engineering controls attempt to design safety into the tools and workspace organization. An example is high-efficiency particulate air filtration systems **FIGURE 4-3**.
   - Personal respiratory protective equipment is used by the employee to prevent exposure to potentially infectious air droplet nuclei—for example, a personal respirator (N95 mask).

TB Screening
Who Should Receive TB Screening?

According to the CDC guidelines, health care workers are at increased risk for TB infection and should be provided with TB testing. This testing must be provided at no cost to employees at risk of exposure. The general population of the United States is considered to be at low risk for TB and should not be routinely tested.

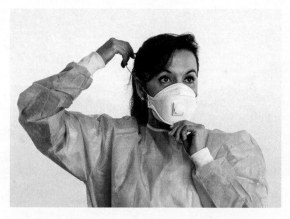

FIGURE 4-3 Wear an N95 or higher respirator when providing care to a suspected or confirmed airborne pathogen patient.
© Andy Sotiriou/Stockbyte/Getty Images.

Frequency of testing for health care workers is based on their risk classification and current infection rates within the community. Two-step testing is recommended for adults who will be retested periodically, such as health care workers and nursing home residents. The two-step process consists of administration of an initial TST or T-IGRA test followed by an additional TST 1 to 3 weeks later. Two-step testing is recommended for health care workers who have not had a TST in the past 12 months. People whose first TST is negative and subsequent test is positive should be evaluated for LTBI. People whose first TST and subsequent test are negative are classified as not infected with TB.

What Is the TB Skin Test?

The TST of choice is the Mantoux test, which uses an intradermal injection of purified protein derivative (PPD). There are three strengths of PPD available; intermediate strength PPD (five tuberculin units) is the standard test material.

A skin test is done by injecting a very small amount of PPD just under the skin (usually the forearm is used). A small bleb (bump) will be raised **FIGURE 4-4**. The bleb will disappear. The injection site is then checked for reaction by your clinician about 48 to 72 hours later. If you fail to have the injection site evaluated in 72 hours and no induration (swelling) is present, the TST will need to be repeated.

What Types of Reactions Occur?

Induration, the hard and bumpy swelling at the injection site, is used for determining a reaction to the PPD. Results are best understood when the general health and risk of exposure to active TB cases are considered in the assessment. The injection site may also be red, but that does not determine a reaction to the PPD or indicate a positive result. Refer to the interpretation guidelines of the American Thoracic Society–CDC advisory panel to assess the measured induration at the injection site.

What Does a Positive Result Mean?

A positive skin test means an infection with *M. tuberculosis* has occurred but does not prove the individual has TB. Referral for further medical evaluation is required to determine a diagnosis of TB disease. People found to have TB disease must be provided effective treatments. The employer provides these treatments to the employee if the illness is found to be work related.

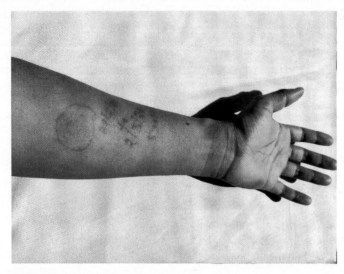

FIGURE 4-4 Positive result of Mantoux test.
© Ashish Kumar/iStock/Getty Images Plus/Getty Images.

Possible False-Negative Results

If a person has had close contact with someone who has TB disease and has a negative reaction to the first skin test, they should be retested about 10 weeks after the last exposure to the person with TB disease. The delay between tests should allow enough time for the body's immune system to respond to an infection with *M. tuberculosis*. A second test will result in a positive reaction at the injection site if an infection with *M. tuberculosis* has occurred.

Contraindications to TB Screening

If you have had a positive TB skin test result in the past, it is not recommended that you receive the test again. If you have had the Bacillus Calmette–Guérin vaccine (sometimes used in foreign countries), you should not have a TB skin test, because it will be positive.

Pregnancy does not exclude a person from being tested. Many pregnant workers have been tested for TB without documented harm to the fetus. You should consult with your physician if you are pregnant and have any questions about receiving a TB skin test.

Meningitis

Meningitis is defined as inflammation of the protective membranes (meninges) covering the brain and spinal cord.

Viruses and bacteria, as well as fungi and other organisms, can cause meningitis. The bacterial form of meningitis is highly contagious and exponentially more serious than viral meningitis. Viral meningitis is more common than any other form of meningitis in most populations. One vaccine currently available can prevent four variants of meningococcal (bacterial) disease. Several other routine vaccinations given in the United States may help prevent other causes of meningitis, both bacterial and viral.

Route of Transmission

Transmission occurs through direct contact and airborne (droplet) routes.

Incubation Period

The incubation period is approximately 2 to 10 days.

Susceptibility

Anyone is susceptible to meningitis. Vaccination for common causes of meningitis provides a significant level of protection for most people. Infants and toddlers are at highest risk for bacterial meningitis and its complications. Other high-risk groups include people with compromised immune systems, preteens and adolescents, and people living in close quarters with others, such as those staying in dormitories or military barracks.

Clinical Presentation

- Fever
- Nausea and vomiting
- Petechial rash (tiny red or purple spots)
- Stiff neck
- Photophobia (light sensitivity)
- Headache
- Altered mental status

Postexposure Treatment

Treatment modalities are dependent on the type of meningitis. General postexposure management guidelines apply. Treatment is symptomatic and may include early use of antibiotics.

Prevention and Control

Airborne precautions should be utilized until the cause is determined not to be bacterial. For nonbacterial forms of meningitis, standard and droplet precautions are sufficient. Vaccination following exposure may provide some protection.

Pertussis

Pertussis (whooping cough) is a highly communicable bacterial respiratory infection caused by the bacterium *Bordetella pertussis*. People of all ages may be affected, but children and infants are at higher risk for serious complications. Pertussis can be recognized by a characteristic paroxysmal whooping cough that may be followed by vomiting. This characteristic "whoop" may not always be present, especially in adults. A sputum test may be needed to confirm diagnosis.

Route of Transmission

Transmission occurs from person to person through droplet and aerosol spread, along with direct contact with the infected secretions or mucous membranes of infected people.

Incubation Period

The average incubation period is 9 to 10 days (range, 6 to 20 days).

Susceptibility

Unimmunized people are at highest risk for contracting pertussis.

Clinical Presentation

- Shortness of breath
- Hypoxia
- Muscle aches
- Fevers
- Runny nose
- Body aches
- Seizures
- Pneumonia
- Cough
- Apnea (cessation of breathing) in infants

Postexposure Treatment

An antibiotic, such as erythromycin, may be administered to lessen the severity of symptoms.

Prevention and Control

Vaccination is available to prevent this disease. People exposed to an active case of pertussis may be offered antibiotics to prevent the development of the disease. Standard and transmission-based precautions should be implemented in all suspected or confirmed cases.

Varicella (Chickenpox)

Chickenpox is a highly contagious disease caused by the varicella-zoster virus. Most cases of chickenpox occur in children younger than 15 years, and the disease is most commonly seen in the spring.

FYI

Reactivation of dormant varicella virus may cause a condition known as herpes zoster or shingles, which causes painful rash and a variety of other symptoms. The rash tends to follow certain regions on the skin known as dermatomes in a readily identifiable pattern. Individuals with herpes zoster can infect others who have never had or been vaccinated for varicella.

Shingles causes numbness, itching, and severe pain, which are followed by a cluster of blisters that appear in a strip. Shingles more commonly appear in people older than 50 years. Cases of shingles have occurred as a result of vaccination, and these cases are seen in a younger population than those that occur after naturally occurring chickenpox. Shingles may persist for months, and even if the rash resolves, persistent pain known as postherpetic neuralgia may occur. Antiviral medication may be used to help treat patients with shingles. Your health care provider determines whether the use of an antiviral medication or any other medication is required. Fever persisting for more than 4 days requires evaluation by a health care provider. Avoid the use of aspirin for symptom relief. Instead, use nonaspirin medications, such as acetaminophen, to relieve pain and fever as instructed by your health care provider.

Route of Transmission

Varicella may be transmitted via direct contact (touching of vesicles) or exposure to airborne droplets or aerosolized particles that are released into the air by the infected person by coughing and/or sneezing.

Transmission by indirect contact can occur by coming in contact with particles recently contaminated by vesicles or mucous membrane discharge from an infected person.

Incubation Period

The incubation period is approximately 10 to 21 days but may be longer in immunocompromised people.

Susceptibility

Anyone not protected by vaccination is susceptible. The disease is usually more severe in adults than in children. Infection usually confers lifelong immunity.

Clinical Presentation

- Fever
- Malaise
- Itchy rash of blisterlike sores

The rash appears as fluid-filled blisters, first appearing on the trunk and face, then spreading to other areas **FIGURE 4-5**. The virus can be transmitted for up to 5 days before the appearance of the rash and will remain transmittable until the lesions have crusted over. Serious complications from the disease may include secondary bacterial infection, pneumonia, or encephalitis (inflammation of the brain).

Postexposure Treatment

If the exposed person is vaccinated, report exposure and watch for signs of infection for a minimum of 21 days. If the exposed person is not immunized and has no history of previous chickenpox, perform serologic testing. If serologic testing is negative, vaccination should be offered to the employee. Vaccination should be administered as soon as possible, within 3 days and up to 5 days after exposure. If infection subsequently develops, the person may be treated with antiviral medications depending on disease severity. For susceptible exposed persons for whom vaccine is contraindicated (immunocompromised or pregnant), provide varicella-zoster immune globulin as soon as possible after exposure and within 10 days.

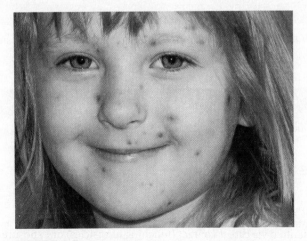

FIGURE 4-5 Chickenpox rash.
© Teo/Shutterstock.

Prevention and Control

Although a vaccine for varicella is available, a vaccinated person still has a 15% to 20% chance of development of a mild form of the disease following exposure. After a single episode of varicella, there is usually lifelong immunity from future outbreaks. It is possible for people to have a second infection of varicella; however, it is generally milder. Standard, contact, and airborne precautions should be used for the treatment of patients with chickenpox.

Measles

Measles is a viral disease that is highly contagious, with a 90% chance of contracting the disease if a person is exposed and not immune. The measles virus is found in the mucus of the nose and throat of an infected person. The virus can live on fomites for up to 2 hours. According to the CDC, in recent years, the United States has seen an increase in measles infections, primarily because of unvaccinated individuals. It is estimated that 140,000 deaths worldwide are attributed to measles annually, with approximately 500,000 cases occurring each year. The actual number of cases is likely much higher due to underreporting. Measles is well controlled in the United States following a brief resurgence in the early 1990s and again in 2019. Most recent cases in the United States are linked to unvaccinated travelers arriving to the United States from measles-prone areas and US residents traveling abroad and then returning to communities with low vaccination rates.

Route of Transmission

Transmission occurs by airborne and aerosol droplets expelled during breathing, coughing, and/or sneezing.

Incubation Period

The incubation period ranges from 7 to 21 days, with the average being approximately 14 days. A person is considered infectious 4 days prior to and 4 days after the onset of a rash.

Susceptibility

Immunocompromised and nonimmunized people are at highest risk for contracting measles.

> **FYI**
>
> In addition to a respiratory protection program, California requires an Aerosol Transmissible Diseases Exposure Control Plan.

> **FYI**
>
> Measles is still a significant cause of vaccine-preventable deaths in pediatrics worldwide.

Clinical Presentation

- Fever
- Runny nose
- Rash (3 to 5 days after respiratory symptoms and fever starts)
- Cough
- Red, watery eyes (conjunctivitis)

- General malaise
- White spots with blue centers (Koplik spots) inside the mouth
- Ear infection (1 out of 10)
- Pneumonia (1 out of 20)
- Encephalitis (1 out of 1,000)

Postexposure Treatment

Measles vaccination given 72 hours prophylactically may prevent disease. Immunoglobulin may provide temporary protection or alter disease severity if given within 6 days after exposure.

Prevention and Control

Vaccination is available to prevent this disease. Standard and airborne transmission precautions should be implemented in all suspected or confirmed cases.

Mumps

Mumps is a vaccine-preventable viral disease. The virus is well controlled following the development of a vaccine in 1948, which has been updated several times and is now combined with measles, rubella, and varicella vaccines in the same dose. During most years, there are typically several hundred cases of mumps in the United States. In the past two decades, there have been a number of notable mumps outbreaks involving several hundred to several thousand individuals.

Route of Transmission

Transmission occurs by respiratory droplets, direct contact, or fomites. It is rapidly spread in susceptible people in close quarters, such as classrooms, military posts, dormitories, or the workplace.

Incubation Period

The incubation period ranges from 14 to 25 days.

Susceptibility

Immunocompromised and nonimmunized people are at highest risk for contracting mumps.

Clinical Presentation

- Unilateral or bilateral facial swelling (jaws and neck)
- Muscle aches
- General malaise
- Headache
- Fever
- Earache
- Tenderness on palpation of facial area
- Meningitis
- Stiff neck
- Encephalitis
- Testicular inflammation
- Ovarian inflammation (may mimic appendicitis)

- Pancreatitis (inflammation of the pancreas)
- Myocarditis (inflammation of the myocardium)
- Kidney inflammation
- Deafness

Postexposure Treatment

Postexposure prophylaxis is based on symptoms. Vaccination is recommended for those people who have not been vaccinated or whose immunization status is unknown.

Prevention and Control

Vaccination is available to prevent this disease. Standard and droplet precautions should be implemented in all suspected or confirmed cases.

Rubella

Rubella is a vaccine-preventable viral disease, sometimes referred to as German measles. This disease is especially harmful to pregnant women. Rubella can cause a variety of birth defects, including deafness, developmental delay, internal organ damage, cataracts, and heart abnormalities.

Route of Transmission

Transmission occurs through airborne contact or through droplets from respiratory secretions of infected people. In addition, infections can occur by direct contact with infected people or fomites contaminated with nasopharyngeal secretions.

Incubation Period

The incubation period ranges from 12 to 23 days, with an average of 14 days. A person should be considered infectious from 7 days prior to the onset of the rash to 7 days after onset.

Susceptibility

Immunocompromised and nonimmunized people are at highest risk for contracting rubella.

Clinical Presentation

- Enlarged, tender lymph nodes
- Muscle aches (especially joints)
- General malaise
- Headache
- Fever
- Stuffy or runny nose
- Inflamed, red eyes
- Pink rash beginning on the face and then spreading to trunk and extremities

Postexposure Treatment

Postexposure prophylaxis is supportive and is combined with medical surveillance. Vaccination is recommended for those people who have not been vaccinated or whose immunization status is unknown.

Prevention and Control

Vaccination is available to prevent this disease. Standard and transmission-based precautions should be implemented in all suspected or confirmed cases.

Hantavirus

Hantavirus is a virus for which there is no available vaccine. Currently, no person-to-person transmission has occurred. This virus first gained national media attention in 1993 when an outbreak occurred in the southwest United States. The virus is not isolated to the United States and has occurred in other parts of the world, including China and Russia. Although there has been no person-to-person transmission, occupational exposure can occur in areas that have a high incidence of deer, mice, and rodent droppings. Rural departments must be especially vigilant in their housekeeping activities. Many agencies have instituted Hantavirus cleaning procedures. In August 2010, a state park employee died as a result of occupational exposure to Hantavirus in Bodie (California) State Historic Park.

Route of Transmission

Infection occurs when someone inhales the Hantavirus. The virus becomes aerosolized when rodent urine and droppings that are contaminated with the virus are disturbed and dispersed in the air. In addition, the disease can be contracted through contact transmission by touching droppings, urine, or nesting materials. There have been a few cases where the virus was transmitted via a bite from a mouse or rat.

Incubation Period

The incubation period ranges from 1 to 6 weeks, with an average of 7 to 14 days.

Susceptibility

Anyone is susceptible to infection by Hantavirus.

Clinical Presentation

- Fever
- Muscle aches
- Headache
- Chills
- Nonproductive cough
- Nausea and vomiting
- Diarrhea
- Abdominal pain
- Dizziness
- Dyspnea
- Tachypnea
- Tachycardia

Postexposure Treatment

There is no vaccine or specific treatment. Medical surveillance and symptomatic treatment are currently the only treatment modalities.

Prevention and Control

Adoption of Hantavirus safety precautions and cleaning protocol includes the following:

- Provide training concerning transmission, prevention, and control.
- Wear vinyl, nitrile, or rubber gloves when cleaning up rodent droppings.
- Use eye protection such as goggles, respirator, and protective clothing while working in environments where Hantavirus dust may be present.
- When possible, clean contaminated equipment or station furniture outside.
- For areas that have been contaminated indoors, urine and droppings should be disinfected with an Environmental Protection Agency-registered disinfectant or a 10% bleach solution to neutralize the virus. Leave for 10 minutes.
- Wipe up the soiled area with disposable towels and place in the trash.
- Ensure that areas such as tables, countertops, drawers, and cabinets around the affected location are disinfected frequently.
- Buildings with heavy rodent infestation may require the use of an agency specially trained in this type of cleanup.

Site-Specific Work Page

Employee Training

Respiratory protection at the worksite: _____

The person at my facility who does fit testing is: _____

At my worksite, masks and respirators are available at the following locations:

_____

Examples of times that I should consider using respiratory protection are:

A. _____

B. _____

C. _____

Limitations to the effectiveness of a respirator include:

A. _____

B. _____

PREP KIT

Vital Vocabulary

coronavirus disease 2019 (COVID-19) The respiratory disease caused by the SARS-CoV-2 virus. This virus primarily affects the lungs and can lead to respiratory failure and death.

Hantavirus An acute viral disease characterized by fever and flulike symptoms progressing to respiratory compromise. Currently, the virus has a greater than 50% mortality rate. Primarily spread by inhalation of airborne particles of urine, feces, and saliva of infected rodents. Other known transmission routes include indirect or direct contact with fomites contaminated with urine, saliva, or fecal droppings or eating contaminated food.

influenza A viral illness that is easily spread from person to person and primarily affects the respiratory system.

measles An acute, highly contagious viral disease characterized by rashes, fever, and respiratory symptoms. Primarily transmitted by respiratory route. Disease can remain active and contagious for up to 2 hours on fomites.

meningitis An inflammation of the meninges, which covers the brain and spinal cord. It is usually caused by a virus or a bacterium.

mumps An acute, highly contagious viral disease characterized by headache, fever, and swelling of salivary glands. Primarily spread through droplets and/or saliva expelled from the nose, mouth, and throat of an infected person. In addition, mumps is secreted in urine, which can be a possible source of transmission.

pertussis (whooping cough) An airborne bacterial infection that primarily affects children younger than 6 years. Patients are feverish and often exhibit a "whoop" sound on inspiration after a coughing attack.

petechial rash A rash consisting of tiny red or purple spots that indicate bleeding within the skin.

rubella An acute, highly contagious viral disease characterized by fever and rashes. Primarily spread via airborne and droplet transmission from respiratory secretions shed by an infected person.

shingles A viral infection caused when the varicella-zoster virus (chickenpox) becomes active in the body after lying dormant, often for decades. Shingles causes numbness, itching, and severe pain, followed by a cluster of blisters that appear in a strip.

tuberculosis (TB) A chronic bacterial disease caused by *Mycobacterium tuberculosis* that usually affects the lungs, but can also affect other organs, such as the brain and kidneys.

Check Your Knowledge

1. The same virus causes chickenpox and shingles.
   - **A.** True
   - **B.** False

2. Flu causes approximately 36,000 deaths each year in the United States.
   - **A.** True
   - **B.** False

3. Pertussis is a vaccine-preventable disease.
   - **A.** True
   - **B.** False

4. COVID-19 first appeared in China in 2019.
   - **A.** True
   - **B.** False

5. Tuberculosis is a serious and often fatal disease if left untreated.
   - **A.** True
   - **B.** False

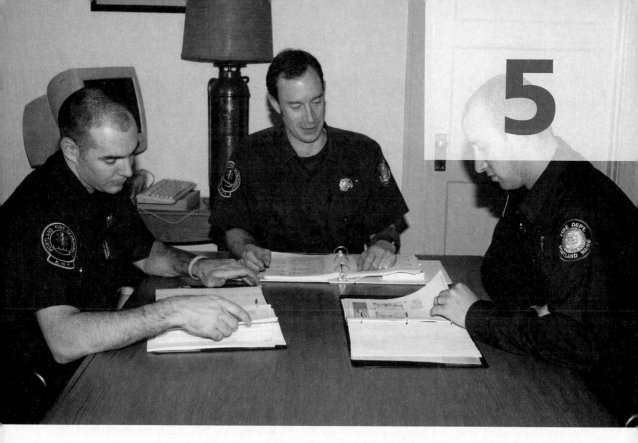

Postexposure Management

Overview

Prevention strategies previously discussed in this manual are intended to reduce or prevent occupational exposure to pathogens. Implementation of these prevention strategies is your best defense against pathogen transmission. However, when these prevention strategies fail, both employers and employees must have a plan detailing postexposure management procedures in order to mitigate any further harm that could occur from the exposure. This plan is known as the exposure control plan. Employers are required by the Occupational Safety and Health Administration (OSHA) to train employees to their specific exposure control plans **FIGURE 5-1**.

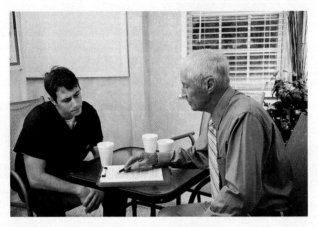

FIGURE 5-1 All employees must be made aware of an employer's exposure control plan.
© Pamela Moore/E+/Getty Images.

What Is an Exposure Control Plan?

The exposure control plan exists as a guideline for employees to know what to do when an exposure occurs. You do not have time to determine what to do *during* an exposure event. A well-documented exposure control plan resolves most of the questions that might arise about an exposure. In addition, the exposure control plan is a key provision of the OSHA Bloodborne Pathogens Standard (29 CFR 1910.1030). A requirement of the plan is for the employer to identify the people who should receive training, protective equipment, vaccination, and other protections of the Standard.

The exposure control plan will contain (at a minimum) the following items:

1. Determination of employee exposure. The exposure determination shall contain a list of all job classifications in which employees have the potential for occupational exposure. The employer shall create a list of all tasks and procedures where occupational exposure could occur. This exposure determination has to be made without regard to the use of personal protective equipment (PPE).

2. Hierarchy of control and/or prevention methods, including administrative, engineering, and work practice controls, as well as PPE.

3. The schedule and method of implementation for each of the applicable subsections:
   - Methods of compliance
   - Human immunodeficiency virus (HIV), hepatitis B virus (HBV), and hepatitis C virus (HCV) research laboratories and production facilities
   - Hepatitis B vaccination
   - Postexposure management
   - Communication of hazards to employees
   - Record keeping

4. Procedures for evaluating exposure incidents, including route(s) of exposure and circumstances under which the exposure incident occurred **FIGURE 5-2**.

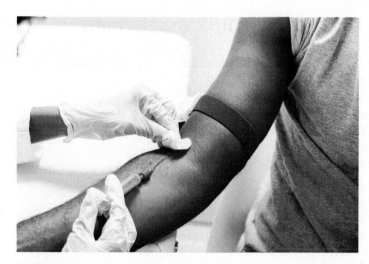

FIGURE 5-2 All procedures that involve the risk of occupational exposure must be outlined in the exposure control plan.
© Andrey_Popov/Shutterstock.

The exposure control plan is required to be reviewed and updated at least annually and whenever necessary to reflect new or modified tasks and procedures that affect occupational exposure and to reflect new or revised employee positions with occupational exposure. The reviews and updates of such plans also must do the following:

- Reflect changes in technology that eliminate or reduce exposure to bloodborne pathogens.
- Document consideration and implementation of appropriate commercially available and effective safer medical devices designed to eliminate or minimize occupational exposure.

General Postexposure Management Steps

OSHA defines an exposure as "a specific eye, mouth, other mucous membrane, nonintact skin, or parenteral contact with blood or other potentially infectious materials (OPIMs) that results from the performance of an employee's duties." The purpose of having an exposure plan is to reduce the likelihood that the exposure will result in infection, which may lead to serious and permanent employee harm. Variable factors influence whether an exposure results in an actual infection. These variable factors are addressed by postexposure management steps—whether general, as listed in this section, or specific, as outlined in your particular employer's plan.

Treat Exposure Site

If the exposure is percutaneous (eg, a needlestick), wash the exposed area with soap and water as soon as possible after the exposure. Do not use any caustic substances or disinfectants (eg, bleach). Do not squeeze the wound site. Mucosal exposure to an area such as the eyes or mouth requires the area to be flushed with copious amounts of water.

Complete Postexposure Risk Assessment

After an exposure, the employee must be given the opportunity to be evaluated by a qualified health care professional. The evaluation will determine what further follow-up and treatment may be recommended. These factors include but are not limited to:

1. Type of exposure
   - Percutaneous injury (depth, extent)
   - Mucous membrane exposure
   - Nonintact skin exposure
   - Bites resulting in blood or OPIM

2. Type and amount of fluid and/or tissue
   - Blood
   - OPIMs

3. Infection status of source
   - HBV positive
   - HCV positive
   - HIV positive

4. Susceptibility of exposed person
   - Hepatitis B vaccination status

Manage Disease

Treatment modalities are disease specific and may include further baseline evaluation and testing, post-exposure prophylaxis, and follow-up testing and counseling. Prompt initiation of postexposure prophylaxis requires immediate reporting and access to an appropriate health care provider.

Complete Postexposure Documentation

Documentation should include:

- Date and time of exposure
- Exposure circumstance
- Type of device involved (if applicable)
- Route of exposure
- Body substance involved
- Volume and duration of contact (estimated)
- Source information
- Information about exposed personnel

Medical records are to be maintained for each employee with occupational exposure in accordance with 29 CFR 1910.1020, "Access to Employee Exposure and Medical Records." These confidential records are to be kept for at least the duration of employment plus 30 years and maintained separately from routine medical records.

Employee medical records are provided upon request of the employee or to anyone having written consent of the employee within 15 working days. Such requests should be sent to the individual identified in your exposure control plan.

Maintaining your own personal record of all exposures and pertinent documents is highly recommended in case of future legal or medical issues resulting from the exposure.

Psychologic Effects

Consider the potential psychologic effect of a high-risk occupational exposure. The employee may experience anger, guilt, embarrassment, fear, anxiety, and myriad other possible emotional responses following an exposure to many bloodborne and airborne pathogens. Many exposures have the possibility of profoundly affecting not just the employee but their families and partners as well. Illness following an occupational exposure may have catastrophic implications for the affected employee, including the possibility of lifelong disease or even death. Consider offering an employee assistance program or similar resources to the employee if available.

Maintain Medical Surveillance

Depending on the type of exposure, further medical treatment and medical surveillance may be warranted. Medical counseling may be an ongoing process to decide treatment and surveillance options if an infection progresses. Depending on the exposure details, the employee may be advised to refrain from the following:

- Donating blood, plasma, or organs
- Risky sexual practices and other behaviors
- Pregnancy and/or breastfeeding

If applicable, patient care responsibilities may need to be modified for the exposed employee to prevent secondary transmission to other employees or patients.

The health care provider should counsel the employee regarding the specific signs and symptoms to watch for, as some diseases develop over a long period of time.

PREP KIT

Vital Vocabulary

medical surveillance A periodic, comprehensive review of an employee's health status as it relates to potential exposures to hazardous agents.

Check Your Knowledge

1. Exposure control plans are not necessary because you would have time to determine what to do during an exposure event.

   A. True

   B. False

2. A hard copy of the plan must be made available to an employee who requests it within _____ days.

   A. 3

   B. 5

   C. 10

   D. 15

3. The exposure control plan must include the procedure for evaluating the circumstances surrounding exposure incidents.

   A. True

   B. False

Sample Exposure Control Plan

This sample plan is provided as a guide to assist in complying with 29 CFR 1910.1030, the Occupational Safety and Health Administration's (OSHA) Bloodborne Pathogens Standard. It is not intended to supersede the requirements detailed in the Standard. Employers should review the Standard for particular requirements that are applicable to their specific situations. It should be noted that this model program does not include provisions for human immunodeficiency virus (HIV) and hepatitis B virus (HBV) laboratories and research facilities that are addressed in section (e) of the Standard. Employers operating these laboratories must include provisions as required by the Standard. Employers will need to add information relevant to their particular facilities in order to develop an effective, comprehensive exposure control plan (ECP). Employers should note that the ECP is expected to be reviewed at least on an annual basis and updated when necessary.

Bloodborne Pathogens Exposure Control Plan

Facility name: _____

Date of original preparation: _____Latest revision: _____

Program Administration

_____ (name of responsible person or department) is/are responsible for the implementation of the ECP.

_____ (name of responsible person or department) will maintain, review, and update the ECP at least annually and whenever necessary to include new or modified tasks and procedures. Contact location and/or phone number: _____.

Those employees who are determined to have occupational exposure to blood or other potentially infectious materials (OPIMs) must comply with the procedures and work practices outlined in this ECP.

_____ (name of responsible person or department) will maintain and provide all necessary personal protective equipment (PPE), engineering controls (eg, sharps containers), labels, and red bags as required by the Standard.

_____ (name of responsible person or department) will ensure that adequate supplies of the aforementioned equipment are available in the appropriate sizes. Contact location and/or phone number: _____.

_____ (name of responsible person or department) will be responsible for ensuring that all medical actions required are performed and that appropriate employee health and OSHA records are maintained. Contact location and/or phone number: _____ _____.

_____ (name of responsible person or department) will be responsible for training, documenting the training, and making the written ECP available to employees, OSHA, and National Institute for Occupational Safety and Health (NIOSH) representatives. Contact location and/or phone number: _____.

Exposure Control Plan

Employees covered by the Bloodborne Pathogens Standard receive an explanation of this ECP during their initial training session. It will also be reviewed in their annual refresher training. All employees have an opportunity to review this plan at any time during their work shifts by contacting _____ (name of responsible person or department). If requested, we will provide an employee with a copy of the ECP free of charge and within 15 days of the request.

_____ (name of responsible person or department) is responsible for reviewing and updating the ECP annually or more frequently if necessary to reflect any new or modified tasks and procedures that affect occupational exposure and to reflect new or revised employee positions with occupational exposure.

In accordance with the OSHA Bloodborne Pathogens Standard, 29 CFR 1910.1030, the following ECP has been developed.

1. Exposure Determination

OSHA requires employers to perform an exposure determination concerning which employees may incur occupational exposure to blood or OPIMs. The exposure determination is made without regard to the use of PPE (ie, employees are considered to be exposed even if they wear PPE). This exposure determination is required to list all job classifications in which all employees may be expected to incur such occupational exposure, regardless of frequency. At this facility, the following job classifications are in this category: _____.

In addition, OSHA requires a listing of job classifications in which some employees may have occupational exposure. Because not all employees in these categories would be expected to incur exposure to blood or OPIMs, tasks or procedures that would cause these employees to have occupational exposure must also be listed in order to understand clearly which employees in these categories are considered to have occupational exposure. The job classifications and associated tasks for these categories are as follows:

Job Classification	**Tasks and Procedures**
_____	_____
_____	_____
_____	_____

2. Implementation Schedule and Method

OSHA also requires that this plan include a schedule and method of implementation for the various requirements of the Standard.

Compliance Methods

Standard precautions will be observed at this facility in order to prevent contact with blood or OPIMs. All blood or OPIMs will be considered infectious regardless of the perceived status of the source individual.

Engineering and work practice controls will be used to eliminate or minimize exposure to employees at this facility. Where occupational exposure remains after institution of these controls, PPE shall also be used. At this facility, the following engineering controls will be used: _____ (list controls, such as sharps containers).

These controls will be examined and maintained on a regular schedule. The schedule for reviewing the effectiveness of the controls is as follows: _____ (list schedule, such as daily or once per week, as well as who is responsible for reviewing the effectiveness of the individual controls, such as the supervisor for each department).

Handwashing facilities are also available to the employees who incur exposure to blood or OPIMs. OSHA requires that these facilities be readily accessible after incurring exposure. At this facility, handwashing facilities are located _____ (list locations, such as patient rooms, procedure area, etc.). If handwashing facilities are not feasible, the employer is required to provide either an antiseptic cleanser with paper towels or antiseptic towelettes. If these alternatives are used, then the hands are to be washed with soap and running water as soon as feasible.

Employers who provide an alternative to readily accessible handwashing facilities should list the location, tasks, and responsibilities to ensure maintenance and accessibility of these alternatives.

After removal of personal protective gloves, employees shall wash hands and any other potentially contaminated skin area immediately or as soon as feasible with soap and water.

If employees incur exposure to their skin or mucous membranes, then those areas shall be washed or flushed with water as appropriate as soon as feasible after contact.

Needles   Contaminated needles and other contaminated sharps will not be bent, recapped, removed, sheared, or purposely broken. OSHA allows an exception to this if the procedure would require that the contaminated needles be recapped or removed and no alternative is feasible and the action is required by the medical procedure. If such action is required, then the recapping or removal of the needle must be done by the use of a mechanical device or a one-handed technique. At this facility, recapping or removal is only permitted for the following procedures: _____ (list the procedures and also list either the mechanical device to be used or, alternatively, if a one-handed technique will be used).

Containers for Reusable Sharps   Contaminated sharps that are reusable are to be placed immediately, or as soon as possible, after use into appropriate sharps containers. At this facility, the sharps containers are puncture resistant, labeled with a biohazard label, and leakproof. (Employers should list here where sharps containers are located as well as who has responsibility for removing sharps from containers and how often the containers will be checked to remove the sharps.)

Location(s):_____

Person/people responsible for checking/changing:_____

Frequency of checking/changing:_____

Work Area Restrictions   In work areas where there is a reasonable likelihood of exposure to blood or OPIMs, employees are not to eat, drink, apply cosmetics or lip balm, smoke, or handle contact lenses. Food and beverages are not to be kept in refrigerators, freezers, shelves, cabinets, or countertops or benchtops where blood or OPIMs are present.

Mouth pipetting or suctioning of blood or OPIMs is prohibited.

All procedures will be conducted in a manner that will minimize splashing, spraying, splattering, and generation of droplets of blood or OPIMs. Methods to accomplish this goal at this facility are _____ (list methods, such as covers on centrifuges or usage of dental dams if appropriate).

Specimens   Specimens of blood or OPIMs will be placed in a container that prevents leakage during the collection, handling, processing, storage, and transport of the specimens.

The container used for this purpose will be labeled or color coded in accordance with the require-ments of the OSHA Standard. (Employers should note that the Standard provides for an exemption for specimens from the labeling or color-coding requirement of the Standard provided that the facility uses universal precautions in the handling of all specimens and the containers are recognizable as container specimens. This exemption applies only while the specimens remain in the facility. If the employer chooses to use this exemption, then it should be stated here.)

Any specimens that could puncture a primary container will be placed within a puncture-resistant secondary container. (The employer should list here how this will be carried out—for example, which specimens, if any, could puncture a primary container, which containers can be used as secondary con-tainers, and where the secondary containers are located at the facility.)

If outside contamination of the primary container occurs, the primary container shall be placed within a secondary container that prevents leakage during the handling, processing, storage, transport, or shipping of the specimen.

Contaminated Equipment   Equipment that has become contaminated with blood or OPIMs shall be examined before servicing or shipping and shall be decontaminated as necessary unless the decontami-nation of the equipment is not feasible. (Employers should list here any equipment that cannot be decon-taminated before servicing or shipping.)

Personal Protective Equipment   All PPE used at this facility will be provided without cost to employ-ees. PPE will be chosen based on the anticipated exposure to blood or OPIMs. The protective equipment will be considered appropriate only if it does not permit blood or OPIMs to pass through or reach the employees' clothing, skin, eyes, mouth, or other mucous membranes under normal conditions of use and for the duration of time that the protective equipment will be used.

Protective clothing will be provided to employees in the following manner: _____ _____ (list how the clothing will be provided to employees—for example, who has re-sponsibility for distribution—and also list which procedures would require the protective clothing and the type of protections required. This could also be listed as an appendix to this program. The employer could use a checklist as follows):

Personal Protective Equipment	Task
▪ Gloves	_____
▪ Lab coat	_____
▪ Face shield	_____

- Clinic jacket   _____
- Protective eyewear (with solid side shield)   _____
- Surgical gown   _____
- Leg and shoe covers   _____
- Utility gloves   _____
- Examination gloves   _____
- Surgical or procedural mask   _____
- Other (list other PPE)   _____

All PPE will be cleaned, laundered, and disposed of by the employer at no cost to employees. All repairs and replacements will be made by the employer at no cost to employees.

All garments that are penetrated by blood shall be removed immediately or as soon as feasible. All PPE will be removed before leaving the work area. The following protocol has been developed to facilitate leaving the equipment at the work area: _____ (list where employees are expected to place the PPE on leaving the work area, as well as other protocols).

Gloves shall be worn where it is reasonably anticipated that employees will have hand contact with blood, OPIMs, nonintact skin, and mucous membranes. Gloves will be available from _____ _____ (state location and/or person who will be responsible for distributing gloves). Gloves will be used for the following procedures: _____ (list procedures).

Disposable gloves used at the facility are not to be washed or decontaminated for reuse and are to be replaced as soon as practical when they become contaminated or as soon as feasible if they are torn or punctured or when their ability to function as a barrier is compromised. Utility gloves may be decontaminated for reuse provided that the integrity of the glove is not compromised. Utility gloves will be discarded if they are cracked, peeling, torn, punctured, or exhibit other signs of deterioration or when their ability to function as a barrier is compromised.

Masks in combination with eye protection devices, such as goggles or glasses with solid side shield or chin-length face shield, are required to be worn whenever splashes, spray, splatter, or droplets of blood or OPIMs may be generated and eye, nose, or mouth contamination can reasonably be anticipated. Situations at this facility that would require such protection are as follows: _____ _____.

The OSHA Standard also requires appropriate protective clothing to be used, such as lab coats, gowns, aprons, clinic jackets, or similar outer garments. The following situations require that such protective clothing be worn: _____.

Housekeeping   This facility will be cleaned and decontaminated according to the following schedule: _____ (list area and time).

Decontamination will be accomplished by using the following materials: _____ _____ (list the materials to be used, such as bleach solutions or Environmental Protection Agency–registered germicides). All contaminated work surfaces will be decontaminated after completion of procedures, immediately or as soon as feasible after any spill of blood or OPIMs, as well as at the end of the work shift if surfaces may have become contaminated since the last cleaning. (Employers should add any information concerning the use of protective coverings, such as plastic wrap, that keeps the surfaces free of contamination.)

All bins, pails, cans, and similar receptacles shall be inspected and decontaminated according to the following schedule: _____.

Any broken glassware that may be contaminated will not be picked up directly with the hands. The following procedures will be used: _____.

Labels   The following labeling method(s) is used in this facility:

Equipment	**Label Type (size, color, etc.)**
Job Classification	**Tasks and Procedures**
_____	_____
_____	_____

_____ (name of responsible person or department) will ensure that warning labels are affixed or red bags are used as required if regulated waste or contaminated equipment is brought into the facility. Employees are to notify _____ (name of responsible person or department) if they discover regulated waste containers, refrigerators containing blood or OPIMs, contaminated equipment, etc, without proper labels.

Regulated Waste Disposal   All contaminated sharps shall be discarded as soon as feasible in sharps containers located in the facility. Sharps containers are located in _____ (specify locations of sharps containers).

Regulated waste other than sharps shall be placed in appropriate containers. Such containers are located in _____ (specify locations of containers).

Laundry Procedures   Laundry contaminated with blood or OPIMs will be handled as little as possible. Such laundry will be placed in appropriately marked bags where it was used. Such laundry will not be sorted or rinsed in the area of use.

All employees who handle contaminated laundry will use PPE to prevent contact with blood or OPIMs.

Laundry at this facility will be cleaned at _____ (specify location). (Employers should note here if the laundry is being sent off-site. If the laundry is being sent off-site, then the laundry service accepting the laundry is to be notified, in accordance with section [d] of the Standard.)

Hepatitis B Vaccine All employees who have been identified as having exposure to blood or OPIMs will be offered the hepatitis B vaccine at no cost to the employee. The vaccine will be offered within 10 working days of their initial assignment to work involving the potential for occupational exposure to blood or OPIMs unless the employee has previously had the vaccine or wishes to submit to antibody testing that shows the employee to have sufficient immunity.

Employees who decline the hepatitis B vaccine will sign a waiver that uses the wording in Appendix A of the OSHA Standard.

Employees who initially decline the vaccine but who later wish to have it while still covered under the Standard may then have the vaccine provided at no cost. (Employers should list here who has responsibility for assuring that the vaccine is offered, the waivers are signed, etc. Also, the employer should list who will administer the vaccine.)

Documentation of refusal of the vaccination is kept at _____ (list location or person responsible for this record keeping).

Vaccination will be provided by _____ (list health care professional who is responsible for this part of the plan) at _____ (location).

After hepatitis B vaccinations, the health care professional's written opinion will be limited to whether the employee requires the hepatitis vaccine and whether the vaccine was administered.

Postexposure Evaluation and Follow-Up

When the employee incurs an exposure incident, it should be reported to _____ (list who has responsibility to maintain records of exposure incidents).

All employees who incur an exposure incident will be offered postexposure evaluation and follow-up in accordance with the OSHA Standard. This follow-up will include the following:

- The route of exposure and the circumstances related to the incident will be documented.
- If possible, the source individual and the status of the source individual will be identified. The source individual's blood will be tested (after consent is obtained) for HIV and/or HBV infectivity.
- The source individual's testing results will be made available to the exposed employee with the exposed employee informed about the applicable laws and regulations concerning disclosure of

the identity and infectivity of the source individual. (Employers may need to modify this provision in accordance with applicable local laws on this subject. Modifications should be listed here.)

- The employee will be offered the option of having their blood collected for testing of the employee's HIV and HBV serological status. The blood sample will be preserved for up to 90 days to allow the employee to decide whether the blood should be tested for HIV serological status; however, if the employee decides before that time that testing will or will not be conducted, then the appropriate action can be taken and the blood sample discarded.
- The employee will be offered postexposure prophylaxis in accordance with the current recommendations of the US Public Health Service. These recommendations are currently as follows (these recommendations may be listed as an appendix to the plan).
- The employee will be given appropriate counseling concerning precautions to take during the period after the exposure incident. The employee will also be given information on what potential illness to be alert for and to report any related experiences to appropriate personnel.

The following person(s) has been designated to assure that the policy outlined here is effectively carried out as well as to maintain records related to this policy: _____ (name of responsible person or department).

Interaction With Health Care Professionals

A written opinion shall be obtained from the health care professional who evaluates employees of this facility. Written opinions will be obtained in the following instances:

1. When the employee is sent to obtain the hepatitis B vaccine.
2. Whenever the employee is sent to a health care professional after an exposure incident.

   Health care professionals shall be instructed:

1. To limit their opinions as to whether the hepatitis B vaccine is indicated and, if so, to ensure that the employee has received the vaccine or has been evaluated following an incident.
2. To ensure that the employee has been informed of the evaluation results.
3. To ensure that the employee has been told about any medical conditions resulting from exposure to blood or OPIMs (note that the written opinion to the employer is not to reference any personal medical information).

Employee Training

All employees who have occupational exposure to bloodborne pathogens receive training conducted by _____ (name of responsible person or department). (Attach a brief description of the individual's qualifications.)

All employees who have occupational exposure to bloodborne pathogens receive training on the epidemiology, symptoms, and transmission of bloodborne pathogen diseases. In addition, the training program covers, at a minimum, the following elements:

1. A copy and explanation of the Standard.

2. An explanation of our ECP and how to obtain a copy.

3. An explanation of methods to recognize tasks and other activities that may involve exposure to blood and OPIMs, including what constitutes an exposure incident.

4. An explanation of the use and limitations of engineering controls, work practices, and PPE.

5. An explanation of the types, uses, location, removal, handling, decontamination, and disposal of PPE.

6. An explanation of the basis for PPE selection.

7. Information on the hepatitis B vaccine, including information on its efficacy, safety, method of administration, the benefits of being vaccinated, and that the vaccine will be offered free of charge.

8. Information on the appropriate actions to take and people to contact in an emergency involving blood or OPIMs.

9. An explanation of the procedure to follow if an exposure incident occurs, including the method of reporting the incident and the medical follow-up that will be made available.

10. Information on the postexposure evaluation and follow-up that the employer is required to provide for the employee following an exposure incident.

11. An explanation of the signs and labels and/or color coding required by the Standard and used at this facility.

12. An opportunity for interactive questions and answers with the person conducting the training session.

    Training materials for this facility are available at _____(list location).

Record Keeping

Annual Review The ECP shall be reviewed and updated at least annually and whenever necessary to reflect new or modified tasks and procedures that affect occupational exposure and to reflect new or revised employee positions with occupational exposure. The review and update of such plans shall also:

1. Reflect changes in technology that eliminate or reduce exposure to bloodborne pathogens.

2. Document annually consideration and implementation of appropriate commercially available and effective safer medical devices designed to eliminate or minimize occupational exposure.

Employee Input The ECP identifies and documents the process by which the employer solicits input from nonmanagerial employees responsible for direct patient care who are potentially exposed to injuries from contaminated sharps in the identification, evaluation, and selection of effective engineering and work practice controls.

Sharps Injury Log   A sharps injury log is established, maintained, and consistently reviewed for recording of percutaneous injuries from contaminated sharps. The sharps injury log is maintained in such a way as to ensure that information concerning the injured employee remains confidential.

The sharps injury log must contain, at a minimum, the following:

1. The type and brand of device involved in the incident.
2. The department or work area where the exposure incident occurred.
3. An explanation of how the incident occurred.

Training Records   Training records are completed for each employee upon completion of training. These documents will be kept for at least 3 years at _____ (name of responsible person or location of records).

The training records include the following:

- The dates of the training sessions.
- The contents or a summary of the training sessions.
- The names and qualifications of the people conducting the training.
- The names and job titles of all the people attending the training sessions.

Employee training records are provided upon request to the employee or the employee's authorized representative within 15 working days. Such requests should be addressed to _____ (name of responsible person or department).

Medical Records   Medical records are maintained for each employee with occupational exposure in accordance with 29 CFR 1910.20, "Access to Employee Exposure and Medical Records."

_____ (name of responsible person or department) is responsible for maintenance of the required medical records. These confidential records are kept at _____ (list location) for at least the duration of employment plus 30 years.

Employee medical records are provided upon request of the employee or to anyone having written consent of the employee within 15 working days. Such requests should be sent to _____ (name of responsible person or department and address).

OSHA Record Keeping   An exposure incident is evaluated to determine if the case meets OSHA's Record-keeping Requirements (29 CFR 1904). This determination and the recording activities are done by _____ (name of responsible person or department).

Appendix B

Hepatitis B Vaccine Declination Form

Appendix A to Section 1910.1030—Hepatitis B Vaccine Declination (Mandatory)

I understand that because of my occupational exposure to blood or other potentially infectious materials, I may be at risk of acquiring hepatitis B virus (HBV) infection. I have been given the opportunity to be vaccinated with hepatitis B vaccine, at no charge to myself; however, I decline the hepatitis B vaccination at this time. I understand that by declining this vaccine, I continue to be at risk of acquiring HBV, a serious disease. If in the future I continue to have occupational exposure to blood or other potentially infectious materials and want to be vaccinated with hepatitis B vaccine, I can receive the vaccination series at no charge to me.

Employee signature: _____

Date: _____

Employer signature: _____

Date: _____

Appendix C

Resources

Bioterrorism	
Centers for Disease Control and Prevention (CDC)	http://emergency.cdc.gov/bioterrorism/
National Institutes of Health (NIH)	www.nlm.nih.gov/medlineplus/biodefenseandbioterrorism.html
Occupational Safety and Health Administration (OSHA)	www.osha.gov/SLTC/bioterrorism/index.html
Bloodborne Pathogens	
OSHA	www.osha.gov/SLTC/bloodbornepathogens/
CDC	www.cdc.gov/niosh/topics/bbp/genres.html
COVID-19 (SARS-CoV-2 virus)	
CDC	https://www.cdc.gov/coronavirus/2019-ncov/index.html
NIH	https://www.nih.gov/coronavirus
Ebola Virus Disease	
CDC	https://www.cdc.gov/vhf/ebola/index.html
World Health Organization (WHO)	https://www.who.int/csr/disease/ebola/en/
Hand Hygiene	
CDC	http://www.cdc.gov/handhygiene/
Hantavirus	
CDC	www.cdc.gov/ncidod/diseases/hanta/hps/
OSHA	www.osha.gov/SLTC/hantavirus/index.html
Hepatitis (A, B, and C)	
CDC	www.cdc.gov/hepatitis/
NIH	www.nlm.nih.gov/medlineplus/hepatitis.html
American Liver Foundation (Diseases of the Liver)	https://liverfoundation.org/for-patients/about-the-liver/diseases-of-the-liver/
American Liver Foundation (Hepatitis A)	https://liverfoundation.org/for-patients/about-the-liver/diseases-of-the-liver/hepatitis-a/
American Liver Foundation (Hepatitis B)	https://liverfoundation.org/for-patients/about-the-liver/diseases-of-the-liver/hepatitis-b/
American Liver Foundation (Hepatitis C)	https://liverfoundation.org/for-patients/about-the-liver/diseases-of-the-liver/hepatitis-c/

continues

(continued)

HIV/AIDS	
CDC	www.cdc.gov/hiv/
US Department of Health and Human Services (HHS)	https://www.hiv.gov/hiv-basics
NIH	www.nlm.nih.gov/medlineplus/hivaids.html
Infection Control and Prevention	
CDC (Eye Protection)	www.cdc.gov/niosh/topics/eye/eye-infectious.html
CDC (Respirators)	www.cdc.gov/niosh/topics/respirators/
CDC (Protective Clothing)	www.cdc.gov/niosh/topics/protclothing/
CDC (Health Care-Associated Infections)	www.cdc.gov/hai/
CDC (Respiratory Hygiene)	www.cdc.gov/flu/professionals/infectioncontrol/resphygiene.htm
Measles	
CDC	www.cdc.gov/vaccines/vpd-vac/measles/default.htm
Meningitis	
CDC	www.cdc.gov/meningitis/index.html
Methicillin-Resistant *Staphylococcus aureus* (MRSA)	
CDC	www.cdc.gov/niosh/topics/mrsa/
Mumps	
CDC	www.cdc.gov/vaccines/vpd-vac/mumps/default.htm
Pertussis	
CDC	www.cdc.gov/pertussis/
NIH	www.nlm.nih.gov/medlineplus/ency/article/001561.htm
Postexposure Management	
University of California, San Francisco	https://nccc.ucsf.edu/clinician-consultation/pep-post-exposure-prophylaxis/
CDC	https://www.cdc.gov/hiv/risk/pep/index.html
Respiratory Protection	
OSHA	www.osha.gov/SLTC/respiratoryprotection/index.html
Rubella	
CDC	www.cdc.gov/vaccines/vpd-vac/rubella/default.htm
Seasonal Influenza	
CDC	www.cdc.gov/flu/
OSHA (Pandemic Flu)	https://www.osha.gov/SLTC/pandemicinfluenza/index.html

Tuberculosis	
CDC and National Institute for Occupational Safety and Health	www.cdc.gov/niosh/topics/tb/
CDC	www.cdc.gov/tb/
OSHA	www.osha.gov/SLTC/tuberculosis/index.html
Vaccinations	
Immunization Action Coalition	www.immunize.org/
CDC (Links to Topics)	www.cdc.gov/vaccines/default.htm
CDC (Vaccine Information Sheets)	http://www.cdc.gov/vaccines/hcp/vis/index.html
Varicella (Chickenpox)	
CDC	www.cdc.gov/vaccines/vpd-vac/varicella/default.htm
Vector-Borne Diseases	
CDC	http://www.cdc.gov/ncezid/dvbd/index.html
West Nile Virus	
CDC	www.cdc.gov/ncidod/dvbid/westnile/index.htm
OSHA	https://www.osha.gov/dts/shib/shib082903b.html

Appendix D

Answer Key

Chapter 1

1. Drawing blood, transporting blood, housekeeping in a health care facility
2. A
3. A
4. B
5. B
6. B

Chapter 2

1. B
2. A
3. A
4. B
5. B
6. A
7. A
8. B
9. B

Chapter 3

1. C
2. A
3. Jaundice, fever, fatigue, loss of appetite, nausea and vomiting, abdominal pain, gray stool, joint pain
4. A
5. A
6. A
7. A
8. A
9. A
10. A
11. A

Chapter 4

1. A
2. A
3. A
4. A
5. A

Chapter 5

1. B
2. D
3. A

acquired immunodeficiency syndrome (AIDS): A collection of signs and symptoms that results from human immunodeficiency virus.

administrative controls: Standard operating procedures and policies that prevent exposures. These include developing training programs, enforcing exclusion of ill employees, implementing respiratory hygiene/cough etiquette strategies, promoting and providing vaccinations, and developing exposure control plans.

airborne pathogens: Disease-causing agents that spread infection through mechanisms such as droplets or dust.

antibodies: Specialized immunity proteins that bind to an antigen to make it more visible to the immune system.

antigen: A substance that causes antibody formation.

blood: The term *blood* refers to human blood, human blood components (which include plasma, platelets, and serosanguinous fluids), and medications derived from blood (such as immunoglobulins, albumin, and clotting factors VIII and IX).

bloodborne pathogens: Disease-causing microorganisms that are carried in human blood or other potentially infectious materials. These pathogens include, but are not limited to, hepatitis B virus, hepatitis C virus, and human immunodeficiency virus.

contaminated sharps: Any contaminated object that can penetrate the skin including, but not limited to, needles, scalpels, broken capillary tubes, and exposed ends of dental wires.

coronavirus disease 2019 (COVID-19): The respiratory disease caused by the SARS-CoV-2 virus. This virus primarily affects the lungs and can lead to respiratory failure and death.

decontamination: The use of physical or chemical means to remove, inactivate, or destroy bloodborne pathogens on a surface or item to the point where they are no longer capable of transmitting infectious particles and the surface or item is rendered safe for handling, use, or disposal.

Ebola virus disease (EVD): A viral infection that causes profound body fluid loss, hemorrhage, and is frequently fatal. This virus typically originates in West Africa but has the ability for widespread transmission as people travel.

engineering controls: Techniques for removal or isolation of a workplace hazard through technology. An airborne infection isolation room, a protective environment, engineered sharps injury prevention devices, and sharps containers are examples of engineering controls.

exposure incident: A specific eye, mouth, mucous membrane, nonintact skin, or parenteral contact with blood or other potentially infectious materials that results from the performance of an employee's duties.

fomites: Inanimate objects, such as desks, faucets, or doorknobs, that have been contaminated with pathogens.

hand hygiene: A general term that applies to any one of the following: (1) handwashing with plain (nonantimicrobial) soap and water; (2) antiseptic handwash (soap containing antiseptic agents and water); (3) antiseptic hand rub (waterless antiseptic product, most often alcohol-based, rubbed on all hand surfaces); or (4) surgical hand antisepsis (antiseptic hand wash or antiseptic hand sanitizer performed preoperatively by surgical personnel to eliminate transient hand flora and reduce resident hand flora).

handwashing facilities: These include alcohol sanitizer dispensers, sinks with soap and hand-drying supplies, or other Centers for Disease Control and Prevention-approved facilities.

Hantavirus: An acute viral disease characterized by fever and flulike symptoms progressing to respiratory compromise. Currently, the virus has a greater than 50% mortality rate. Primarily spread by inhalation of airborne particles of urine, feces, and saliva of infected rodents. Other known transmission routes include indirect or direct contact with fomites contaminated with urine, saliva, or fecal droppings or eating contaminated food.

hepatitis B virus (HBV): A virus that causes liver infection. It ranges in severity from a mild illness lasting a few weeks (acute) to a serious long-term (chronic) illness that can lead to liver disease or liver cancer.

hepatitis C virus (HCV): A virus that causes liver infection. HCV infection sometimes results in an acute illness but most often becomes a chronic condition that can lead to cirrhosis of the liver and liver cancer.

hepatitis: Inflammation of the liver.

human immunodeficiency virus (HIV): A virus that infects immune system blood cells in humans and renders them less effective in preventing disease.

immunity: Resistance to an infectious disease.

immunization: A process or procedure by which resistance to an infectious disease is produced in a person.

influenza: A viral illness that is easily spread from person to person and primarily affects the respiratory system.

jaundice: A yellowing of the skin associated with hepatitis infection.

measles: An acute, highly contagious viral disease characterized by rashes, fever, and respiratory symptoms. Primarily transmitted by respiratory route. Disease can remain active and contagious for up to 2 hours on fomites.

medical surveillance: A periodic, comprehensive review of an employee's health status as it relates to potential exposures to hazardous agents.

meningitis: An inflammation of the meninges, which covers the brain and spinal cord. It is usually caused by a virus or a bacterium.

mucous membrane: An area of the body, other than the skin, that is exposed to the outside environment. These areas have specialized epithelial cells that prevent pathogens and other materials from entering the body. Mucous membranes include the respiratory tract, digestive tract, urinary tract, vagina, eyes, and inside of the ear.

mumps: An acute, highly contagious viral disease characterized by headache, fever, and swelling of salivary glands. Primarily spread through droplets and/or saliva expelled from the nose, mouth, and throat of an infected person. In addition, mumps is secreted in urine, which can be a possible source of transmission.

needleless systems: Devices that do not utilize needles for (1) the withdrawal of body fluids after initial venous or arterial access is established, (2) the administration of medication or fluids, and (3) any other procedure involving the potential for occupational exposure to bloodborne pathogens due to percutaneous injuries from contaminated sharps.

occupational exposure: Reasonably anticipated skin, eye, mucous membrane, or parenteral contact with blood or other potentially infectious materials (OPIMs) that may result from the performance of an employee's duties. "Reasonably anticipated contact" includes, among others, contact with blood or OPIMs (including regulated waste) as well as incidents of needlesticks.

opportunistic infections: Illnesses caused by various organisms, many of which often do not cause disease in people with healthy immune systems.

other potentially infectious material (OPIM): Fluids such as semen, vaginal secretions, cerebrospinal fluid, synovial fluid, pleural fluid, pericardial fluid, peritoneal fluid, amniotic fluid, saliva in dental procedures, any body fluid that is visibly contaminated with blood, and all body fluids in situations where it is difficult or impossible to differentiate between body fluids; any unfixed tissue or organ (other than intact skin) from a live or dead human; any cell and tissue cultures, and human immunodeficiency virus (HIV)- or hepatitis B virus (HBV)-containing culture medium or other solutions; and blood, organs, or other tissues from experimental animals (especially those infected with HIV or HBV).

pandemic: A disease outbreak that spreads across multiple countries or continents.

pathogen: Any microorganism that causes disease.

percutaneous: Occurring through the skin, such as drawing blood with a needle.

personal protective equipment (PPE): A variety of barriers used alone or in combination to protect mucous membranes, skin, and clothing from contact with infectious agents. PPE includes gloves, masks, respirators, goggles, face shields, and gowns.

pertussis (whooping cough): An airborne bacterial infection that primarily affects children younger than 6 years. Patients are feverish and often exhibit a "whoop" sound on inspiration after a coughing attack.

petechial rash: A rash consisting of tiny red or purple spots that indicate bleeding within the skin.

prophylaxis: Protective measures designed to prevent the spread of disease.

regulated waste: Liquid or semiliquid blood or other potentially infectious materials (OPIMs); contaminated items that would release blood or OPIMs in a liquid or semiliquid state if compressed; items that are caked with dried blood or OPIMs and are capable of releasing these materials during handling; contaminated sharps; and pathologic and microbiologic wastes containing blood or OPIMs.

respiratory hygiene/cough etiquette: A combination of measures designed to minimize the transmission of respiratory pathogens via droplet or airborne routes in health care settings.

rubella: An acute, highly contagious viral disease characterized by fever and rashes. Primarily spread via airborne and droplet transmission from respiratory secretions shed by an infected person.

severe acute respiratory syndrome coronavirus 2 (SARS-CoV-2): The virus that causes an infection called coronavirus disease 2019 (COVID-19), which primarily affects the lungs and can lead to respiratory failure and death.

sharps: Any objects used or encountered in the industries covered by subsection (a) of the Occupational Safety and Health Administration Bloodborne Pathogens Standard that can be reasonably anticipated to penetrate the skin or any other part of the body and to result in an exposure incident. These objects include, but are not limited to, needle devices, scalpels, lancets, broken glass, broken capillary tubes, exposed ends of dental wires and dental knives, drills, and burs.

sharps injury: Any injury caused by a sharp, including, but not limited to, cuts, abrasions, or needlesticks.

sharps injury log: A written or electronic record satisfying the requirements of subsection (c)(2) of the Occupational Safety and Health Administration Bloodborne Pathogens Standard.

shingles: A viral infection caused when the varicella-zoster virus (chickenpox) becomes active in the body after lying dormant, often for decades. Shingles causes numbness, itching, and severe pain, followed by a cluster of blisters that appear in a strip.

source individual: Any individual, living or dead, whose blood or other potentially infectious materials may be a source of occupational exposure to the employee. Examples include, but are not limited to, hospital and clinic patients; clients in institutions for the developmentally disabled; trauma patients; clients of drug and alcohol treatment facilities; residents of hospices and nursing homes; human remains; and people who donate or sell blood or blood components.

standard precautions: A group of infection prevention practices that apply to all patients, regardless of suspected or confirmed diagnosis or presumed infection status.

terminal clean: An intense disinfecting process to kill pathogens and remove organic material from the environment in order to make it safe to use again by other patients, visitors, and health care providers.

transmission-based precautions: Additional steps instituted when routes of transmission are not interrupted by standard precautions alone; that is, contact precautions, droplet precautions, airborne precautions.

tuberculosis (TB): A chronic bacterial disease caused by *Mycobacterium tuberculosis* that usually affects the lungs, but can also affect other organs, such as the brain and kidneys.

vaccine: A suspension of inactive or killed microorganisms administered orally or injected into a human to induce active immunity to infectious disease.

vector: An animal or insect (eg, fleas, mosquitoes, birds, rodents) that transmits pathogens, such as rabies, malaria, or West Nile virus, to human hosts.

work area: The area where work involving risk of exposure or potential exposure to blood or other potentially infectious materials exists, along with the potential contamination of surfaces.

work practice controls: Controls that reduce the likelihood of exposure by altering the manner in which a task is performed (eg, prohibiting recapping of needles by a two-handed technique and use of patient handling techniques).

Index